Leukotrienes

New Concepts and Targets for Therapy

Leukotrienes
New Concepts and Targets for Therapy

Edited by

DR IAN RODGER,[1] DR JACK BOTTING[2]
and PROF. SVEN-ERIK DAHLÉN[3]

[1] *Merck Frosst Canada, Inc., Pointe-Claire-Dorval, Quebec, Canada*
[2] *The William Harvey Research Institute, Saint Bartholomew's Hospital Medical College, London, United Kingdom*
[3] *Asthma and Allergy Research, Institute of Environmental Medicine, Karolinska Institutet, Stockholm, Sweden*

*Proceedings of a conference held
on June 12–13, 1997
in London, UK, supported by an educational grant from*

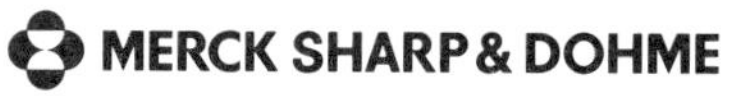

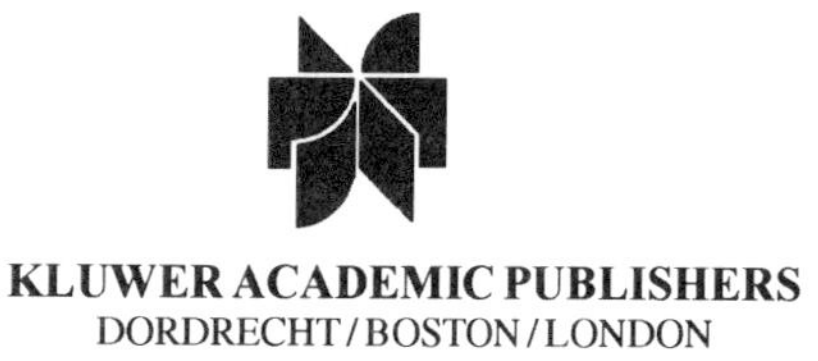

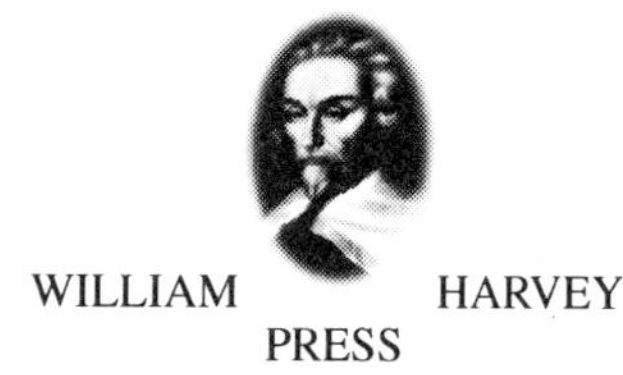

01-2003 SGA 97-W-6094-B
This material is provided as a professional service to the medical profession by Merck Sharp & Dohme. The views expressed in this publication reflect the experience and opinion of the authors and not necessarily those of Merck Sharp & Dohme. The prescribing information from the Company (manufacturer) for any product described in this publication should be consulted prior to prescribing.

Distributors

---

for North, Central and Latin America: Kluwer Academic Publishers, PO Box 358, Accord Station, Hingham, MA 02018–0358, USA
for all other countries: Kluwer Academic Publishers Group, Distribution Center, PO Box 322, 3300 AH Dordrecht, The Netherlands

A catalogue record for this book is available from the British Library

ISBN 0–7923–8738–4

Copyright

Published in the United Kingdom by Kluwer Academic Publishers, PO Box 55, Lancaster, UK, and William Harvey Press, The Medical College, Charterhouse Square, London EC1M 6BQ, UK.

Printed in Great Britain.

Contents

List of Contributors

N. C. Barnes
The London Chest Hospital, Bonner Road, London E2 9JX, UK
Co-author: A. Macfarlane

C. Brink
CNRS Centre Chirurgical Marie Lannelongue, 133 ave de la Résistance,
92350 Le Plessis Robinson, France
Co-author: J.-P. Gascard

S.-E. Dahlén
Experimental Asthma and Allergy Research, Institute of Environmental Medicine,
PO Box 210, Karolinska Institutet, S-171 77 Stockholm, Sweden

P. R. Devchand
Institut de Biologie Animale, Bâtiment de Biologie, Université de Lausanne,
Lausanne, CH-1015, Switzerland
Co-author: W. Wahli

A. Ford-Hutchinson
Merck Frosst Centre for Therapeutic Research, 16711 Trans Canada Highway,
Kirkland, Quebec H9H 3L1, Canada
Co-author: P.-J. Jakobsson

P. Howarth
Southampton General Hospital, Tremona Road, Southampton SO9 4XY, UK

J. Kips
Department of Respiratory Diseases, University Hospital Ghent, De Pintelaan 185,
B 9000 Belgium
Co-author: R. Pauwels

M. Kumlin
Experimental Asthma and Allergy Research, Institute of Environmental Medicine,
PO Box 210, Karolinska Institutet, S-171 77 Stockholm, Sweden

T. H. Lee
Department of Allergy and Respiratory Medicine, 4th Floor, Hunt's House,
Guy's Hospital, London SE1 9RT, UK
Co-author: B. E. A. Lams

S. Nicosia
Institute of Pharmacological Sciences, University of Milan, Via Balzaretti 9, 20133 Milan, Italy
Co-authors: E. Rovati, V. Capra, S. Ravasi, M. Mezzetti, T. Viganò,
M. R. Accomazzo, A. Hernandez, A. Bonazzi, M. Bolla, E. Galbiati, M. Di Luca,
A. Caputi, A. M. Villa, S. Esposito, S. Doglia, M. Rovelli and G. Folco

M. Peters-Golden
Pulmonary and Critical Care Medicine Division, 6301 MSRB III, Box 0642, University of Michigan Medical School, Ann Arbor, MI 48109, USA

K. F. Rabe
Krankenhaus Grosshansdorf, Wöhrendamm 80, D-22927 Grosshansdorf, Germany

A. Sala
Center for Cardiopulmonary Pharmacology, University of Milan, Via Balzaretti 9, 20133 Milan, Italy

G. Santoro
Institute of Experimental Medicine, CNR, Viale K. Marx 15/43, 00137 Roma, and Department of Biology, University of Rome Tor Vergata, Via della Ricerca Scientifica, 00133 Roma, Italy

A. Szczeklik
Jagellonian University School of Medicine, Department of Medicine, Skawińska 8, 31–066 Kraków, Poland
Co-author: M. Sanak

Preface

In the two decades since the elusive "slow reacting substance of anaphylaxis" (SRS-A) was identified as a product of the action of the 5-lipoxygenase enzyme on arachidonic acid, it has been well established that the leukotrienes are key mediators of both allergy and inflammation. Their release by allergen or other challenge has been demonstrated in the lungs of asthmatic subjects, and measurement of urinary leukotriene concentrations in such patients has been shown to be a valuable, non-invasive indicator. Significant progress has been made towards the characterization of the leukotriene receptor subtypes, exemplified by the cloning of the LTB_4 receptor earlier this year. Coupled with this there has been a continued elucidation of signal transduction mechanisms underlying receptor activation. Consequent upon these advances has been the development of potent antagonists of the $CysLT_1$ receptor, and both these and inhibitors of leukotriene biosynthesis have entered clinical practice in the therapy of asthma. In this clinical setting antagonists of the $CysLT_1$ receptor have been shown to be an effective therapy in chronic asthmatics, against antigen- and exercise-induced bronchoconstriction, and in aspirin-intolerant asthmatics. The advent of this new class of agents promises to change the way in which asthmatic patients are currently treated.

Research into the intercellular distribution of those enzymes involved in the biosynthesis of leukotrienes, and a variety of additional pharmacological studies, have raised the possibility that transcellular synthesis occurs, whereby cells containing leukotriene C_4 synthase (such as endothelial cells) can utilize substrate produced by circulating leukocytes to form cysteinyl-leukotrienes. Such observations could have profound pathological significance in certain cardiovascular inflammatory disorders. Similarly, techniques enabling the determination of the precise intracellular location of phospholipase, 5-lipoxygenase and 5-lipoxygenase activating protein (FLAP) have clearly established that leukotriene biosynthesis occurs at the level of the nuclear envelope. This information, taken together with the identification of intranuclear receptors for leukotrienes, suggests that these lipid mediators might have markedly extended biological roles via intranuclear actions.

The evidence attesting to the pivotal role played by leukotrienes in a variety of pathophysiological settings is clear and convincing. With the continued elucidation of the molecular and biochemical events surrounding the leukotrienes it is also apparent that further clinical applications of biosynthesis inhibitors and/or receptor antagonists are likely. It is the purpose of this monograph to bring together authoritative review articles of the advances in this rapidly changing area, written by international authorities in the field of leukotriene research.

1 Molecular mechanisms of leukotriene synthesis: the changing paradigm

M. PETERS-GOLDEN

Leukotrienes (LTs) are potent lipid mediators which modulate a multitude of fundamental intracellular processes. While their pathophysiological role has been best established in asthma, they are probably important participants in many other disease processes characterized by inflammation, cellular proliferation, and fibrogenesis. They also subserve a homoeostatic role in antimicrobial host defence[1]. In view of the actions and importance of LTs, substantial effort over the last several years has been directed at increasing our understanding of their synthesis. The purpose of this brief chapter will be to review these recent advances in LT synthesis, with an emphasis on the biochemistry, molecular biology and cell biology of the key enzymes involved.

OVERVIEW OF THE LEUKOTRIENE SYNTHETIC PATHWAY

Leukotriene synthesis can be triggered by a variety of soluble and particulate stimuli, including antigens, microbes, cytokines, immune complexes and model agonists such as calcium ionophores. These result in the activation of signal transduction cascades and the generation of second messengers such as Ca^{2+}, which in turn activate phospholipase A_2 (PLA_2). This enzyme initiates LT synthesis by catalysing the hydrolysis of arachidonic acid (AA) from membrane phospholipids. Although there are multiple isoforms of PLA_2, the most attractive candidate to subserve this function is cytosolic PLA_2 ($cPLA_2$), a Ca^{2+}-dependent and AA-preferring 85 kDa enzyme[2].

The liberated free AA can then be acted on by the first committed enzyme in the LT synthetic pathway, 5-lipoxygenase (5-LO). This 78 kDa protein catalyses a two-step reaction: oxygenation of AA at carbon 5 to form an unstable intermediate, 5-hydroperoxyeicosatetraenoic acid (5-HPETE), followed by dehydration of 5-HPETE to yield the epoxide leukotriene A_4 (LTA_4). Maximal activity of 5-LO requires Ca^{2+}, ATP, and hydroperoxide, and its efficient utilization of endogenously released AA in intact cells requires a 18 kDa helper protein, termed 5-LO activating protein (FLAP). FLAP is an AA-binding protein which is thought to optimally 'present' substrate to 5-LO. LTA_4 is the precursor for the stable bioactive LTs. It can be hydrolysed by LTA_4 hydrolase to LTB_4, which has potent chemotactic and leukocyte-activating effects, or conjugated with reduced glutathione by LTC_4 synthase to yield LTC_4; LTC_4 can be further modified extracellularly by sequential amino acid removal to yield LTD_4 and LTE_4. Collectively, LTC_4, D_4 and E_4 are known as the cysteinyl LTs, and comprise the smooth muscle contractile and vascular permeability activities long recognized as slow-reacting substance. Examination of this pathway thus identifies several critical proteins which are potential loci for regulation of LT synthesis[3], as will be discussed.

CELLULAR SOURCES OF LEUKOTRIENES

Phospholipase A_2s, including $cPLA_2$, are ubiquitously expressed among various cell types. However, 5-LO and FLAP proteins are largely restricted to cells of bone marrow origin (myeloid cells), and it is these cell types which have the greatest capacity for LT generation. Interestingly, the LT synthetic capacity of members of one family of myeloid cell, the resident tissue macrophage, varies in a tissue-specific fashion. In particular, pulmonary alveolar macrophages have a far greater LT synthetic capacity than do macrophages from other tissues[4]. In addition, the profile of LTs synthesized, which is dictated by a cell's complement of distal LT synthases, varies with the cell type. Thus, eosinophils and mast cells synthesize predominantly LTC_4, while neutrophils synthesize predominantly LTB_4. Macrophages synthesize a mixture of LTC_4 and LTB_4, with differences depending primarily on species; rat and human macrophages produce predominantly LTB_4, while murine macrophages produce predominantly LTC_4.

Although the LT synthetic capacity of structural or parenchymal cells (epithelial cells, endothelial cells, fibroblasts, smooth muscle cells) is minuscule relative to myeloid cells, they can generate LTs under some circumstances, and even these low levels of LTs can play important biological roles[5]. The distal LT synthase enzymes (LTA_4 hydrolase and LTC_4 synthase) are expressed somewhat more widely than are 5-LO and FLAP, being found in a variety of cell types which lack the latter. Parenchymal cells can also, therefore, contribute to LT production by converting LTA_4 released by myeloid cells to either LTB_4 or LTC_4, a process known as 'transcellular' LT synthesis[6].

REGULATION OF LEUKOTRIENE SYNTHESIS

Although LTs must be synthesized de novo, this can be accomplished quite rapidly (within several minutes) following addition of an agonist, via activation of enzymes which are constitutively present within cells. Activation of both $cPLA_2$ and 5-LO requires an increase in intracellular Ca^{2+}, and the activity of 5-LO is optimized in the presence of ATP. Neither FLAP nor distal LT synthases depend on an 'activation' event, but LTC_4 synthase requires reduced glutathione as a co-substrate. Thus, even the immediate generation of LTs can be influenced by the intracellular levels of the small molecules Ca^{2+}, ATP and glutathione.

The activities of the LT-synthesizing enzymes can be rapidly augmented by post-translational modifications such as phosphorylation. Phosphorylation of serine 505 on $cPLA_2$, which occurs following the addition of a variety of 'priming' agents, increases the catalytic efficiency with which this enzyme causes hydrolysis of AA[7]. The actions of 5-LO also appear to be augmented by kinase activation[8,9], and there is some evidence for direct phosphorylation of 5-LO[10].

A delayed type of priming or enhancement of LT synthesis occurs with transcriptional or translational events which increase the steady-state level of key enzyme proteins. This phenomenon has been observed for $cPLA_2$ as well as another Ca^{2+}-dependent enzyme, secretory PLA_2. It has also been observed for 5-LO and FLAP, and the regulation of expression of these two proteins will be briefly considered here. The promoter region of the 5-LO gene resembles that of 'housekeeping' genes, in that only a few *cis*-acting elements are present[11]. This is surprising given the restricted cellular and tissue distribution of the encoded protein. Polymorphisms of the 5-LO promoter have recently been described, with mutations resulting in reduced transcription being noted in approximately 35% of individuals[12]; it remains to be determined whether these mutations are associated with diminished LT production or have clinical relevance. In contrast to that for 5-LO, the promoter region of the FLAP gene has multiple regulatory elements[13]. In most experimental systems, FLAP expression is regulated concordantly with 5-LO expression[14], although examples of discordant expression have been described[15,16]. Despite differences in their promoter structures, expression of both proteins has been reported to be upregulated by similar factors; these include various cytokines, glucocorticoids, and models of macrophage differentiation. It is important to note that the regulatory effects of a given agent can vary depending on the cell type. For example, granulocyte-macrophage colony stimulating factor increases the expression of both 5-LO and FLAP proteins in neutrophils[17,18], but increases only the expression of $cPLA_2$ in macrophages[19]. Finally, reduced expression of 5-LO and FLAP has been reported in alveolar macrophages obtained from patients infected with the human immunodeficiency virus[20].

In addition to the concentrations of small molecule co-factors, the steady-state levels of key proteins, and modifications that alter the catalytic activities of these proteins, one further determinant of LT synthesis has recently been recognized: the intracellular compartmentalization of LT-synthesizing proteins. This has been the focus of extensive investigation in our own and other laboratories in recent years, and a number of surprising findings have been revealed. An update on the current state of knowledge in this area will be the subject of the remainder of this chapter.

THE TRANSLOCATION MODEL FOR 5-LIPOXYGENASE ACTIVATION

The intracellular locale of the proteins necessary for LT synthesis went largely unstudied for many years. An important advance in our understanding of the mechanism of 5-LO activation was the demonstration that the enzyme undergoes a Ca^{2+}-dependent redistribution or translocation from its locale within a soluble compartment in resting cells to a membrane compartment following agonist activation[21]. This process of translocation could reasonably be assumed to bring the enzyme in proximity to its membrane-derived substrate. It was soon determined that $cPLA_2$ likewise underwent a Ca^{2+}-dependent redistribution from a soluble to a membrane compartment upon stimulation[22]. Since the helper protein FLAP was also present in the membrane fraction of cells both in the resting and stimulated states[23], a model was formulated in which agonist activation resulted in co-localization of the proteins necessary for arachidonate release and the initiation of LT synthesis. Since LTs were known to be efficiently secreted from cells, the site at which these proteins were co-localized was assumed to be the plasma membrane. However, these early subcellular fractionation studies were not capable of adequately resolving compartmentalization, and there was no a priori reason to do so at the time given the assumptions regarding the primacy of the plasma membrane.

ROLE OF THE NUCLEAR ENVELOPE IN LEUKOTRIENE SYNTHESIS

Surprisingly, when activated blood neutrophils were studied by immunoelectron microscopy, both 5-LO and FLAP were localized to the nuclear envelope[24]. At about the same time, peritoneal macrophages were gently disrupted (so that the plasma membrane but not the nuclear membrane was ruptured) and separated into nuclear, cytosolic, and non-nuclear membrane fractions which were then subjected to immunoblot analysis. FLAP was found predominantly in the nuclear fraction of both resting and stimulated cells; furthermore, 5-LO was found to translocate from the cytosolic to the nuclear fraction upon activation[25]. These results indicating the nuclear envelope to be the site of 5-LO and FLAP co-localization in activated leukocytes appear to reflect a universal phenomenon, now also verified for alveolar macrophages[26,27], blood monocytes[26], mast cells[28], the rat basophilic leukaemia (RBL) mast cell-like cell line[27] and eosinophils (Sporn P, Peters-Golden M, Brock TG, unpublished results). Localization of 5-LO at the nuclear envelope in activated cells has now also been confirmed in situ, since immunohistochemical analysis revealed an increased number of macrophages with this staining pattern in lung sections from patients with idiopathic pulmonary fibrosis, a disease characterized by constitutive overproduction of LTs by alveolar macrophages ex vivo[29]. Of course, these findings with 5-LO and FLAP raised the question of whether $cPLA_2$ translocated to the same membrane. Recent studies using appropriate disruption and fractionation methods as well as immunofluorescence microscopy have indeed revealed that $cPLA_2$ is also localized primarily at the nuclear envelope in a variety of types of stimulated cells[25,30–32]. Importantly, translocation of $cPLA_2$ to the nuclear envelope is associated with selective hydrolysis of nuclear membrane phospholipids[30]. Recently, LTC_4 synthase has been shown to have a high degree of homology with FLAP; like FLAP, it is an integral membrane protein located primarily at the nuclear envelope[33]. Taken together, there is now abundant evidence suggesting that the nuclear envelope is the site at which AA release (at least that mediated by $cPLA_2$), LTA_4 synthesis, and LTA_4 conversion to LTC_4 all occur. The mechanism by which the translocation of $cPLA_2$ and 5-LO which originate in the cytosol is targeted to the nuclear envelope, as opposed to other intracellular membranes, remains to be elucidated. In any case, these findings raise the important question of why mediators destined for extracellular secretion would be synthesized deep within the cell, and this will be considered at the end of this chapter.

CELL-SPECIFIC COMPARTMENTALIZATION OF 5-LIPOXYGENASE IN RESTING CELLS

Initial studies in unstimulated blood neutrophils[34] and peritoneal macrophages[25] demonstrated that 5-LO was predominantly cytosolic, and this finding has been extended to blood monocytes[26] and eosinophils (Sporn P, Peters-Golden M, Brock TG, unpublished results). Unexpectedly, subsequent fractionation as well as immunomicroscopic studies of isolated alveolar macrophages[26,27], mast cell-like RBL cells[34] and primary mast cells[28] revealed abundant intranuclear 5-LO in addition to that found within the cytosol. Importantly, an intranuclear pool of 5-LO in alveolar macrophages has been confirmed in situ by immunohistochemical staining of normal human lung tissue[29]. A proportion of the intranuclear pool in RBL cells is insoluble and has biochemical characteristics suggesting that it is chromatin-associated[34]. Immunoelectron microscopic analysis of human alveolar macrophages demonstrated that intranuclear 5-LO was not randomly distributed, but was instead concentrated in the euchromatin region[26], that portion of the nucleus where actively transcribing genes are distributed. That the intranuclear pool of 5-LO participates in cellular LT synthesis is suggested by the facts that it is catalytically active in cell-free assays and translocates to the nuclear envelope upon agonist stimulation[27]. These findings indicate that compartmentalization of 5-LO in unstimulated cells varies depending on the cell type, with some cells exhibiting exclusively cytosolic enzyme and others containing both cytosolic and intranuclear pools; in either case, activation is associated with translocation to the nuclear envelope. The mechanisms by which compartmentalization of 5-LO is differentially regulated in different cell types are not currently understood.

DYNAMIC REGULATION OF 5-LIPOXYGENASE COMPARTMENTALIZATION

Rather than a static model in which 5-LO compartmentalization is considered to be dictated solely by cell type, several lines of evidence indicate that it is, in fact, a dynamically regulated process even within a given cell type. The first comes from studies with various mononuclear phagocyte populations. Blood monocytes, the precursors for all mature tissue macrophages, contain cytosolic 5-LO[26]. While mature peritoneal macrophages retain this cytosolic distribution[25], alveolar macrophages do not[26,27], indicating that nuclear import of this protein accompanies monocyte migration into the pulmonary alveolar space, but not the peritoneum. Second, the recruitment of blood neutrophils into sites of inflammation (either pulmonary alveolus or peritoneum) is associated with rapid movement of 5-LO into the nucleus, which is not itself accompanied by LT synthesis[35]. This can be mimicked by adherence of blood neutrophils to various surfaces[35]. A similar adherence-dependent movement of 5-LO from cytosol into nucleus has recently been observed with blood eosinophils (Sporn P, Peters-Golden M, Brock TG, unpublished results). A final example involves DMSO-induced differentiation of the promyelocytic leukaemic cell line, HL-60, into granulocytic cells, a process known to be associated with increased expression of both 5-LO and FLAP[36]. We have observed that incubation of these cells with serum results in a shift of 5-LO localization from the cytosol to the intranuclear compartment (Brock TG, Peters-Golden M, unpublished results). Again, the molecular mechanisms by which dynamic nuclear import of 5-LO is mediated are as yet undefined. However, it is interesting that experimental conditions in which nuclear import of both cPLA$_2$[37] and cyclooxygenase-2[38], an inducible form of the enzyme responsible for conversion of AA to prostaglandins, have recently been described.

METABOLIC IMPLICATIONS OF 5-LIPOXYGENASE LOCALIZATION

The fact that 5-LO and FLAP (along with other relevant proteins) are localized to the nuclear envelope of activated cells implies that LT synthesis is initiated at this site. As a result, the local concentrations of LTs within the nucleus are likely to be quite high. Teleologically, these observations suggest that the potential nuclear actions of these lipid mediators may be more important than those extracellular actions which have been classically recognized. The recent identification of a nuclear receptor for LTB_4 supports the contention that LTs exert intranuclear effects[39]. Interestingly, this receptor was a member of the steroid superfamily of transcription factors and its activation was capable of inducing gene transcription. Theoretically, LTs could also modulate nuclear events by interacting directly with nucleic acids, transcription factors or signalling pathways. It should also be recalled that reactive oxygen species are a by-product of arachidonate 5-lipoxygenation, and these reactive intermediates could themselves possess nuclear actions by activating transcription factors or otherwise modifying nuclear constituents.

The propensity of particular LT-forming proteins to be localized at particular intracellular sites raises the possibility that metabolic coupling among proteins will be dictated by their topographic proximity. This notion posits that both the access of 5-LO/FLAP to free AA and their capacity to supply LTA_4 for LT synthesis will be enhanced by the proximity of PLA_2 and LT synthases, respectively, to the nuclear envelope. In this regard, it has long been recognized that different functional pools of AA exist within a given cell type[40], and different metabolic fates for AA could reflect the topographic proximity of PLA_2s and downstream enzymes.

Dynamic nuclear import of 5-LO adds a further measure of complexity to the regulation of LT synthesis. It should be emphasized that nuclear import is not itself associated with LT synthesis. How does this phenomenon in resting cells influence subsequent LT generation upon activation? In two different experimental models (peritoneal *vs* alveolar macrophages and blood *vs* recruited neutrophils), the latter cells with intranuclear 5-LO require a higher dose of ionophore to trigger LT synthesis than do the former cells with cytosolic enzyme[4,35]. This could reflect the likelihood that intranuclear Ca^{2+} concentrations are lower than cytosolic Ca^{2+} concentrations following the addition of an extracellular stimulus. However, alveolar macrophages[4], recruited neutrophils[35] and serum-treated differentiated HL-60 cells (Brock TG, Peters-Golden M, unpublished results), all of which possess intranuclear 5-LO, all display greater maximal capacities for LT production in response to stimuli than do the corresponding cells with cytosolic 5-LO. The lower sensitivity and greater capacity of these cells with an intranuclear distribution of 5-LO could alternatively reflect a lower hydroperoxide tone in the nuclear than cytosolic compartment. In any case, a growing body of evidence indicates that compartmentalization of 5-LO is an important determinant of LT synthetic responses.

NON-METABOLIC IMPLICATIONS OF 5-LIPOXYGENASE LOCALIZATION

The localization of 5-LO could have biological implications apart from its catalytic products, LTs and reactive oxygen species. The 5-LO protein has a Src homology-3 binding motif[41], which could mediate protein–protein interactions between the enzyme and Src homology-3 domains. These domains are typically present in proteins which are substrates for tyrosine phosphorylation, and purified 5-LO has been shown to bind with certain cytoskeletal proteins[41]. This motif on 5-LO has been suggested to mediate enzyme translocation in response to activation[10]. The facts that 5-LO can be found within the euchromatin region of nuclei and can be demonstrated to be chromatin-associated further suggest that the enzyme could likewise interact directly with intranuclear proteins or, perhaps, genes.

CONCLUSIONS

Our understanding of the molecular mechanisms and regulation of LT synthesis has increased dramatically in recent years. In particular, investigations into the cell biology of this metabolic pathway have revealed an unexpected role for the nucleus. While many questions of a molecular and functional nature remain to be answered, this finding provides the impetus to explore novel intracellular actions of LTs beyond those traditionally appreciated.

Acknowledgements

The author gratefully acknowledges the contributions of Drs Thomas Brock, Michael Coffey, Marc Bailie, Jerome Wilborn, Peter Sporn, Robert Paine, John Woods, and Mr Robert McNish to the work discussed herein which was performed in his laboratory.

References

1. Baillie M, Standiford T, Laichalk L, Coffey M, Strieter R, Peters-Golden M. Leukotriene-deficient mice manifest enhanced lethality from Klebsiella pneumonia in association with decreased alveolar macrophage phagocytic and bactericidal activities. J Immunol. 1996; 157: 5221–4.
2. Dennis E. Diversity of group types, regulation, and function of phospholipase A_2. J Biol Chem. 1994; 269: 13057–60.
3. Ford-Hutchinson A, Gresser M, Young R. 5-Lipoxygenase. Annu Rev Biochem. 1994; 63: 383–417.
4. Peters-Golden M, McNish RW, Hyzy R, Shelly C, Toews GB. Alterations in the pattern of arachidonate metabolism accompany rat macrophage differentiation in the lung. J Immunol. 1990; 144: 263–70.
5. Peppelenbosch M, Tertoolen L, den Hertog J, de Laat S. Epidermal growth factor activates calcium channels by phospholipase A_2/5-lipoxygenase-mediated leukotriene C_4 production. Cell. 1992; 69: 295–303.
6. Maciouf J, Fitzpatrick F, Murphy R. Transcellular biosynthesis of eicosanoids. Pharmacol Res. 1989; 21: 1–7.
7. Kramer R, Roberts E, Manetta J, Hyslop P, Jakubowski J. Thrombin-induced

phosphorylation and activation of Ca^{2+}-sensitive cytosolic phospholipase A_2 in human platelets. J Biol Chem. 1993; 268: 26795–804.

8. Liles WC, Meier KE, Henderson WR. Phorbol myristate acetate and the calcium ionophore A23187 synergistically induce release of LTB4 by human neutrophils: Involvement of protein kinase C activation in regulation of the 5-lipoxygenase pathway. J Immunol. 1987; 138: 3396–402.

9. Peters-Golden M, McNish R, Sporn P, Balazovich K. Basal activation of protein kinase C in rat alveolar macrophages: implications for arachidonate metabolism. Am J Physiol: Lung Cell Mol Physiol. 1991; 261: L462–L71.

10. Lepley R, Muskardin D, Fitzpatrick F. Tyrosine kinase activity modulates catalysis and translocation of cellular 5-lipoxygenase. J Biol Chem. 1996; 271: 6179–84.

11. Hoshiko S, Radmark O, Samuelsson B. Characterization of the human 5-lipoxygenase gene promoter. Proc Natl Acad Sci USA. 1990; 87: 9073–7.

12. In Asano K, Beier D, et al. Naturally occurring mutations in the human 5-lipoxygenase gene promoter that modify transcription factor binding and reporter gene transcription. J Clin Invest. 1997; 99: 1130–7.

13. Kennedy B, Diehl B, Boie Y, Adam M, Dixon R. Gene characterization and promoter analysis of the human 5-lipoxygenase-activating protein (FLAP). J Biol Chem. 1991; 266: 8511–16.

14. Reid GK, Kargman S, Vickers PJ, et al. Correlation between expression of 5-lipoxygenase-activating protein, 5-lipoxygenase, and cellular leukotriene synthesis. J Biol Chem. 1990; 265: 19818–23.

15. Jakobsson P, Steinhilber D, Odlander B, Radmark O, Claesson H, Samuelsson B. On the expression and regulation of 5-lipoxygenase in human lymphocytes. Proc Natl Acad Sci USA. 1992; 89: 3521–5.

16. Coffey MJ, Gyetko M, Peters-Golden M. 1,25-Dihydroxyvitamin D3 upregulates 5-lipoxygenase metabolism and 5-lipoxygenase activating protein in peripheral blood monocytes as they differentiate into mature macrophages. J Lipid Mediators. 1993; 6: 43–51.

17. Pouliot M, McDonald P, Khamzina L, Borgeat P, McColl S. Granulocyte-macrophage colony-stimulating factor enhances 5-lipoxygenase levels in human polymorphonuclear leukocytes. J Immunol. 1994; 152: 851–8.

18. Pouliot M, McDonald P, Borgeat P, McColl S. Granulocyte/macrophage colony-stimulating factor stimulates the expression of the 5-lipoxygenase-activating protein (FLAP) in human neutrophils. J Exp Med. 1994; 179: 1225–32.

19. Brock TG, McNish RW, Coffey MJ, Ojo TC, Phare SM, Peters-Golden M. Effect of granulocyte-macrophage colony-stimulating factor on eicosanoid production by mononuclear phagocytes. J Immunol. 1996; 156: 2522–7.

20. Coffey M, Phare S, Kazanjian P, Peters-Golden M. 5-Lipoxygenase metabolism in alveolar macrophages from subjects infected with the human immunodeficiency virus. J Immunol. 1996; 157: 393–9.

21. Rouzer CA, Kargman S. Translocation of 5-lipoxygenase to the membrane in human leukocytes challenged with ionophore A23187. J Biol Chem. 1988; 263: 10980–8.

22. Channon J, Leslie C. A calcium-dependent mechanism for associating a soluble arachidonoyl-hydrolyzing phospholipase A2 with membrane in the macrophage cell line RAW 264.7. J Biol Chem. 1990; 265: 5409–13.

23. Miller DK, Gillard JW, Vickers PJ, et al. Identification and isolation of a membrane protein necessary for leukotriene production. Nature. 1990; 343: 278–81.

24. Woods J, Evans J, Ethier D, et al. 5-Lipoxygenase and 5-lipoxygenase activating protein are localized in the nuclear envelope of activated human leukocytes. J Exp Med. 1993; 178: 1935–46.

25. Peters-Golden M, McNish R. Redistribution of 5-lipoxygenase and cytosolic phospholipase A_2 to the nuclear fraction upon macrophage activation. Biochem Biophys Res Commun. 1993; 196: 147–53.

26. Wood J, Coffey M, Brock T, Singer I, Peters-Golden M. 5-Lipoxygenase is located in the euchromatin of the nucleus in resting human alveolar macrophages and translocates to the nuclear envelope upon cell activation. J Clin Invest. 1995; 95: 2035–40.

27. Brock TG, McNish RW, Peters-Golden M. Translocation and leukotriene synthetic capacity of nuclear 5-lipoxygenase in rat basophilic leukemia cells and alveolar macrophages. J Biol Chem. 1995; 270: 21652–8.

28. Chen X-S, Naumann T, Kurre U, Jenkins N, Copeland N, Funk C. cDNA cloning, expression, mutagenesis, intracellular localization, and gene chromosomal assignment of mouse 5-lipoxygenase. J Biol Chem. 1995; 270: 17993–9.

29. Wilborn J, Bailie M, Coffey M, Burdick M, Strieter R, Peters-Golden M. Constitutive activation of 5-lipoxygenase in the lungs of patients with idiopathic pulmonary fibrosis. J Clin Invest. 1996; 97: 1827–36.

30. Peters-Golden M, Song K, Marshall T, Brock T. Translocation of cytosolic phospholipase A_2 to the nuclear envelope elicits topographically localized phospholipid hydrolysis. Biochem J. 1996; 318: 797–803.

31. Glover S, Bayburt T, Jonas M, Chi E, Gelb M. Translocation of the 85-kDa phospholipase A2 from cytosol to the nuclear envelope in rat basophilic leukemia cells stimulated with calcium ionophore or IgE/antigen. J Biol Chem. 1995; 270: 15359–67.

32. Schievella A, Regier M, Smith W, Lin L. Calcium-mediated translocation of cytosolic phospholipase A_2 to the nuclear envelope and endoplasmic reticulum. J Biol Chem. 1995; 270: 30749–54.

33. Penrose J, Spector J, Lam B, Friend D, Xu K, Jack R, Austen K. Purification of human lung LTC_4 synthase and preparation of a polyclonal antibody. Am J Respr Crit Care Med. 1995; 152: 283–9.

34. Brock TG, Paine R, Peters-Golden M. Localization of 5-lipoxygenase to the nucleus of unstimulated rat basophilic leukemia cells. J Biol Chem. 1994; 269: 22059–66.

35. Brock T, McNish R, Bailie M, Peters-Golden M. Rapid import of cytosolic 5-lipoxygenase into the nucleus of neutrophils after in vivo recruitment and in vitro adherence. J Biol Chem. 1997; 272: 8276–80.

36. Kargman S, Rouzer CA. Studies on the regulation, biosynthesis, and activation of 5-lipoxygenase in differentiated HL60 cells. J Biol Chem. 1989; 264: 13313–20.

37. Sierra-Honigmann M, Bradley J, Pober J. 'Cytosolic' phospholipase A2 is in the nucleus of subconfluent endothelial cells but confined to the cytoplasm of confluent endothelial cells and redistributes to the nuclear envelope and cell junctions upon histamine stimulation. Lab Invest. 1996; 74: 684–95.

38. Coffey R, Hawkey C, Damstrup L, et al. Epidermal growth factor receptor activation induces nuclear targeting of cyclooxygenase-2, basolateral release of prostaglandins, and mitogenesis in polarizing colon cancer cells. Proc Natl Acad Sci USA. 1997; 94: 657–62.

39. Devchand P, Keller H, Peters J, Vazquez M, Gonzalez F, Wahli W. The $PPAR_\alpha$-leukotriene B_4 pathway to inflammation control. Nature 1996; 384: 39–43.

40. Humes J, Sadowski S, Galavage M, Goldenberg M, Subers E, Bonney R, Kuehl F Jr. Evidence for two sources of arachidonic acid for oxidative metabolism by mouse peritoneal macrophages. J Biol Chem. 1982; 257: 1591–4.

41. Lepley RA, Fitzpatrick F. 5-lipoxygenase contains a functional Src homology 3-binding motif that interacts with the Src homology 3 domain of Grb2 and cytoskeletal proteins. J Biol Chem. 1994; 269: 24163–8.

2 Leukotriene receptors

S.-E. DAHLÉN

Drugs which selectively inhibit the formation or action of leukotrienes (LT) have been introduced as a new therapy in asthma. Despite the ongoing delineation of the molecular biology of the enzymes in the LT pathways, corresponding information about the receptors for LTs is sparse. Knowledge of LT receptors is mainly derived from studies of functional responses. The drugs which have been developed as antagonists of tissue receptors for cysteinyl-leukotrienes (cys-LTs) were discovered by classical strategies such as screening of new chemical entities in functional or ligand-binding assays. This chapter will review our current understanding of LT receptors.

LEUKOTRIENE B$_4$

Profile of biological activity

Leukotriene B$_4$ (LTB$_4$) was the first LT discovered[1] when the 5-lipoxygenase pathway in human leukocytes was explored[2]. With the exception of a contractile effect in the guinea-pig lung parenchyma[3–5], inflammatory cells are the principal targets for the biological activity of LTB$_4$ (Table 1). It is a potent stimulus for activation of leukocytes, eliciting chemokinetic and chemotactic responses in vitro[6]. In vivo, LTB$_4$, increases leukocyte rolling and adhesion to the venular endothelium[7]. This initial chemotactic response is followed by emigration of leukocytes into the extravascular space[7]. During a short-lasting exposure to LTB$_4$, mainly polymorphonuclear leukocytes are recruited[8,9]. With prolonged exposure to LTB$_4$, as presumably occurs when LTB$_4$ is formed in vivo, other granulocytes, including eosinophils, are found in tissues or exudates[10]. Accordingly, LTB$_4$ has been shown to be a chemoattractant in interleukin-5 primed eosinophils[11], and to stimulate production of interleukin-5 in T-lymphocytes[12].

In addition to effects on leukocyte recruitment, LTB$_4$ stimulates secretion of superoxide anion and release of various granular constituents from leukocytes[13,14]. Among the effects of LTB$_4$ on inflammatory cells, it may affect expression of low affinity receptors for IgE on B-lymphocyte cell lines[15] and synthesis of IgE induced by interleukin-4[16]. More recently, the observation that LTB$_4$ is an agonist for the nuclear transcription factor peroxisome proliferator-activated receptor α (PPARα) has created considerable interest[17]. The finding may implicate a role for LTB$_4$ in the control of central events in lipid metabolism and inflammation[18]. The structure–activity relationship for this effect of LTB$_4$ and the influence of antagonists of LTB$_4$ on the response have yet to be elucidated, but the observations nevertheless point to the possibility that LTB$_4$ also has intracellular and nuclear targets, which may participate in long-term control of gene expression.

Table 1 Schematic overview of the receptors which appear to mediate different effects of cys-LTs. For effects denoted in bold, the receptor characteristics have been established, whereas the remaining effects need further studies with regard to receptor characteristics. The main endogenous ligands are also shown. As indicated, some, but not all, of the biological effects of lipoxin A_4 are mediated by interaction with $CysLT_1$-receptors [reviewed in Ref. 99]. As discussed in the text, LTE_4 is usually inactive or only weakly active at $CysLT_2$ receptors

Receptor	Agonists	Effects
BLT receptor	LTB_4 20-OH-LTB_4 20-COOH-LTB_4 12R-HETE	**Leukocyte activation** Cytokine secretion IgE synthesis Nuclear transcription ($PPAR_\alpha$)
CysLT₁ receptor	LTC_4 LTD_4 LTE_4 (Lipoxin A_4)	**Bronchospasm** **Plasma exudation** **Vasoconstriction** **Plasma exudation** **Eosinophil recruitment** Mucus secretion Cardiodepression Smooth muscle proliferation
CysLT₂ receptor	LTC_4 LTD_4 (LTE_4)	Vasorelaxation and constriction Smooth muscle contraction

The 5*S*, 12*R*-position of the hydroxyl groups in LTB_4 appears to be critical for biological activity[13,19]. For example, 5*S*-HETE and 5*S*, 12*S*-DHETE are both less potent than LTB_4 in guinea-pig lung parenchyma[3,5,19], and the responses elicited by these compounds are also different with respect to time course and mode of action[3,5]. In contrast, a 5*S*, 12*R*-DHETE with 6-*trans* and 8-*cis* double bonds (LTB_4 is 6-*cis* and 8-*trans* but otherwise has an identical structure) formed by the LTA_4 hydrolase in *Xenopus laevis*, was found to share the mode of action of LTB_4 in guinea-pig lung strips[20].

Receptors for LTB₄

The different profiles of biological activities for LTB_4 and cys-LTs (Table 1) suggested that the two main classes of LTs possessed distinct receptors. Experimental data have indeed established that LTB_4 acts at a specific receptor, now designated the BLT-receptor[21]. Radioligand binding experiments have been useful in the exploration of the properties of BLT-receptors, and specific [³H] LTB_4 binding has been demonstrated in many tissues including human polymorphonuclear leukocytes (PMNs)[22,23]. The binding sites in PMNs are selectively inhibited by guanine nucleotides[24,25] and structurally related metabolites displaced LTB_4 with a potency which correlated with their activities in chemotactic assays[26].

A number of selective and relatively potent antagonists of LTB_4 have been developed[27]. A few compounds have entered into early clinical testing in man, LY-293,

111 (VML 295) probably being the most studied. This particular compound was recently found to inhibit LTB_4-induced neutrophil responses in vivo and allergen-induced PMN activation, but had no effect on allergen-induced early or late phase airway obstruction in asthmatics[28]. The results obtained with LY-293, 111 in asthmatics argue against an important role for LTB_4 as a mediator in asthma, but do not exclude the possibility that LTB_4 may be involved in other pulmonary reactions.

Pharmacological evidence has accumulated to suggest that BLT-receptors are G-protein coupled[24,25], but it was only very recently possible to isolate the cDNA for a BLT-receptor in retinoic acid-differentiated HL-60 cells[29]. The cDNA encoded a 352 amino acid cell-surface protein which was G-protein coupled and mediated chemotaxis. Incidentally, this cDNA had previously been studied, but was then described as an orphan receptor possibly mediating chemoattractant responses[30]. Northern blotting experiments of human tissues displayed a preferential expression of mRNA for the BLT receptor in PMNs[29]. There was also some expression in the spleen and thymus, whereas most other tissues examined, including the lung, showed no or insignificant expression of message for the BLT-receptor[29].

It has been observed that chemotaxis especially is mediated at lower agonist concentrations of LTB_4 than those required for degranulation and superoxide generation[13,22,31]. Ligand binding experiments have also demonstrated the presence of low and high affinity binding sites[22,32]. These observations have been taken as evidence for two subclasses of receptors for LTB_4. However, when tested against competitive antagonists, similar dose ratios are produced for all effects of LTB_4[27]. Likewise, naturally occurring metabolites or synthetic analogues show similar displacement potencies for the low and high affinity binding sites[25]. Therefore, the apparent high and low affinity states may reflect G-protein coupled or uncoupled states of the BLT receptor. There is thus currently no basis for the definition of subclasses of receptors for LTB_4, and the available antagonists appear to block the effects of LTB_4 and its immediate metabolites at a common BLT receptor. However, the recent cloning of the BLT receptor[29] has created the opportunity for new developments in this area.

THE cys-LEUKOTRIENES

Profile of biological activity

The identification of LTC_4 as a slow reacting substance in a mouse mastocytoma cell line[33] sparked the recognition that the slow reacting substance of anaphylaxis (SRS-A) was made up of LTC_4 and its two immediate metabolites LTD_4 and LTE_4[34–41]. This in turn led to research on the biological properties of the cys-LTs along the lines suggested by the original observations on the properties of biologically generated SRS-A[42]. Thus, it was soon documented that in particular LTC_4 and LTD_4 were potent inducers of bronchoconstriction in guinea-pig airways in vitro and in vivo[43,44] and caused contraction of isolated human bronchi[45–47]. When tested in assays which had been used to distinguish SRS-A from other mediators, it was established that LTC_4 and LTD_4 were indeed inactive in systems which were unresponsive to SRS-A, for example rabbit bronchus and rat uterus[48].

When injected intravenously into guinea-pigs, LTC_4 and LTD_4 caused biphasic changes in blood pressure[43,44]. These two cys-LTs also increased Evans' blue accumulation in the skin[43,44], suggesting an increase in microvascular permeability. In the hamster cheek pouch LTC_4 and LTD_4 caused exudation of plasma proteins in postcapillary venules[7]. In addition, LTC_4 and LTD_4 induced arteriolar constriction, but the plasma exudation was not a consequence of this[7]. In guinea-pig, LTC_4, LTD_4 and LTE_4 were each capable of inducing Evans' blue accumulation in the airways[48]. Their effects were observed in all airway segments, from the most peripheral small bronchiole to the trachea, and there was evidence of dye accumulation in superficial as well as deep layers of the airway mucosa.

The biological effects of LTE_4 have generally been studied much less, perhaps because this LT was found to be an incomplete and less potent agonist than LTC_4 and LTD_4 in the guinea-pig ileum[49]. However, LTE_4 has been shown to possess a bronchoconstrictor activity in vitro and in vivo which is very similar to that of LTC_4 and LTD_4[50]. Prolonged exposure to LTE_4 may produce enhancement of the responsiveness of smooth muscle to histamine[51,52]. Moreover, LTE_4 is a full agonist for contraction of human bronchi in vitro[41,53], and was not significantly less potent than LTC_4 and LTD_4[53,54]. Apart from a superfusion study, which found LTE_4 much less potent than LTD_4 in human bronchi[55], investigations using large numbers of tissue specimens and comparable non-flow tissue bath conditions, have consistently found LTE_4 to be either equipotent[53,54] or only slightly less potent than LTD_4 or LTC_4 in human bronchi[56]. Although the kinetics and transduction mechanisms for the individual cys-LTs on human airway smooth muscle need to be characterized more extensively, the contention that LTE_4 as a rule is less bioactive than LTC_4 or LTD_4 should be dismissed.

In addition to the bronchospastic and vasoactive properties of cys-LTs (Table 1) LTC_4 and LTD_4 may stimulate mucus secretion in isolated animal and human airways[57–59]. Experiments in isolated perfused hearts also disclosed a depressant effect on cardiac contractility[60,61]. This effect correlated with coronary vasoconstriction[62], but a direct negative inotropic effect on the myocardium may also be involved[61,63].

More recently, additional effects with potential relevance to the role of cys-LTs in asthma and pulmonary inflammation have been reported. Thus, increased infiltration of eosinophils into the airways mucosa of asthmatics was observed following inhalation of LTE_4[64], and inhalation of LTD_4 increased the number of eosinophils in induced sputum samples from asthmatics[65]. The capacity of cys-LTs to promote eosinophil recruitment has recently been confirmed in experimental models[66,67], although the mechanisms involved remain to be defined. There is also experimental data in vitro[68,69] and in vivo[70] supporting the fact that cys-LTs may be involved in airway smooth muscle proliferation and remodelling.

The spasmogenic and vasoactive properties of cys-LTs, and the effects of LTB_4 on leukocytes and the microcirculation, have been fairly well characterized, whereas the effects of LTs on many other systems have so far received comparatively little attention. There would seem to be many areas where the effects of LTs need to be explored to obtain more information about possible physiological functions and pathogenetic mechanisms. The large variations in responsiveness to LTs between different animal species may provide important clues to the further investigation of LT receptors.

Receptors for cys-leukotrienes

When the SRS-A antagonist FPL 55712 was tested against LTC_4 and LTD_4 in guinea-pig airway preparations[71], it was evident that it was a competitive antagonist of LTD_4 but not LTC_4[43,72,73]. After inhibition of the metabolic conversion of LTC_4 into LTD_4, LTC_4 was as potent an agonist as LTD_4 in the guinea-pig trachea, but the effect of LTC_4 could not be antagonized by FPL 55712[73] or subsequently developed antagonists of LTD_4[74,75]. These observations supported the hypothesis of two different receptors for cys-LTs, tentatively called the LTC_4 and the LTD_4 receptors. The findings with metabolic inhibitors also argued against the hypothesis that LTC_4 was bioactive only after having been transformed into LTD_4[76].

However, when the influence of FPL 55712 on LTC_4 and LTD_4 was examined in human bronchi in the presence of the conversion inhibitor serine borate, it was discovered that FPL 55712 antagonized the effect of LTC_4 and LTD_4 in this tissue to the same extent[54]. The human airways were thus different from the guinea-pig trachea or ileum where LTC_4 and LTD_4 appeared to cause contractions by activation of different receptors. Subsequent studies with more potent antagonists have indeed confirmed that LTC_4 and LTD_4 act at the same receptor in human airways[53,54,77]. Moreover, LTE_4 is also a full and potent agonist at the receptor for cys-LTs in human bronchi[53,54], and a selective antagonist such as ICI-204, 219 (zafirlukast) produces an identical shift in the concentration–response curve for each of LTC_4, LTD_4 and LTE_4[53].

LTC_4 and LTD_4 cause contraction of human pulmonary vessels[46]. When Labat and co-workers examined the effects of antagonists on contractions evoked by cys-LTs in human pulmonary veins[56], they discovered that the responses were resistant to several potent compounds (ICI-198, 615, MK-571 and SKF 104, 353). The agonist sensitivity was also different from the bronchial preparations, LTE_4 being a comparatively weak agonist, producing only a transient submaximal contraction of the human pulmonary vein. Responses to both LTC_4 and LTD_4 which were resistant to the current class of antagonists had previously been reported in animal tissues such as ferret trachea[78], but not received as much attention as the antagonist-resistant effects of LTC_4 in guinea-pig ileum[49] and trachea[75–78]. The findings in the human tissues contributed to the recognition that there seemed to exist at least two different receptors for cys-LTs, one preferentially sensitive to LTC_4 (guinea-pig ileum and trachea) and the other mediating contractions in response to both LTC_4 and LTD_4 (human pulmonary vein and ferret trachea).

The effects of LTC_4 and LTD_4 on the human pulmonary vein are antagonized in an apparently competitive manner by the leukotriene analogue BAY u9773 (5(S)-hydroxy-6(R)-(4'-carboxyphenylthio)-7,9-$trans$-11,14-cis-eicosatetraenoic acid)[56]. BAY u9773 was subsequently found to be a competitive antagonist of atypical responses to LTC_4 or LTD_4 in guinea pig ileum[79] and trachea[80], sheep bronchus[80] and trachea[81] and ferret trachea[80]. However, the compound also antagonizes the effects of cys-LTs in preparations where the responses are sensitive to the currently available antagonists[80]. Therefore, BAY u9773 is not a selective antagonist of atypical responses to cys-LTs, but it has broader, non-selective, properties.

On the basis of the evidence presented, the names *CysLT$_1$* and *CysLT$_2$* have been introduced to describe responses which are sensitive and resistant, respectively, to the class of antagonist drugs currently being introduced in the clinic[21]. As indicated in Table 2, there are tissues such as guinea-pig ileum and trachea where both types of receptors co-exist, and there are tissues which seem to have homogenous populations of receptors. For example *CysLT$_1$* receptors predominate in human bronchi[53,54] and rat lung[80], whereas *CysLT$_2$* receptors appear to dominate in sheep trachea[81]. However, the presence of opposing and interdependent responses to cys-LTs[82] highlight the need to obtain more selective antagonists and agonists.

The current classification of two main classes of receptors for cys-LTs is a first step supported by the available evidence, but is nevertheless likely to be an oversimplification. There is for example a significant difference in the potency of ICI-198, 615 between rat lung and guinea-pig trachea[80], which could reflect species-differences. However, in an early study using the prototype FPL 55712 in the guinea-pig[72], it was shown that the response to LTD$_4$ in the ileum was most susceptible to blockade, whereas the trachea, and in particular the lung parenchyma, required considerably higher concentrations of antagonist. Such differences within the same species have been observed in other studies, and may indicate the presence of subclasses of the receptors. The observation that contraction in response to LTD$_4$ in guinea-pig lung parenchyma is poorly inhibited by both potent *CysLT$_1$* antagonists such as ICI-198, 615 as well as by the combined *CysLT$_1$/CysLT$_2$* antagonist BAY u9773[80] raises the possibility of a third main subclass (*CysLT$_3$*).

Likewise, although differences in metabolism between tissues may contribute to differences in agonist potency and efficacy for the individual cys-LTs, it appears likely that the presence of additional receptor subclasses could also explain several apparently disparate observations. For example, the *CysLT$_2$* responses in guinea-pig ileum or trachea are evoked by LTC$_4$ alone[49,75–77,80] whereas LTC$_4$ and LTD$_4$, and occasionally also LTE$_4$, may cause their effects through activation of putative

Table 2 Summary of the cysLT-receptors and their antagonists. The parenthesis around BAY u9773 as a CysLT$_2$-antagonist has been introduced to indicate that it is a non-selective antagonist with properties of a combined CysLT$_1$/CysLT$_2$ antagonist. As discussed in the text, it is likely that there exist further subclasses of both CysLT$_1$ and CysLT$_2$ receptors

	CysLT$_1$	*CysLT$_2$*
Tissue:	Human bronchus Guinea-pig trachea and ileum Guinea-pig gall bladder Rat lung strip	Human pulmonary artery and vein Guinea-pig trachea and ileum Sheep trachea and bronchus Ferret trachea
Antagonist:	FPL 55712, LY 171,883 ICI 198, 615/ICI 204,219, MK-571/MK-679/MK-476, SKF 104, 353/SKF 106,203 ONO 1078/SB 205,312, RG 12,525, CGP 45715 BAY x7195,(BAY u9773)	(BAY u9773)

$CysLT_2$ receptors in sheep trachea[83] and human pulmonary vein[56]. Conversely, LTC_4 appears inactive at the $CysLT_1$ receptor in guinea-pig trachea and ileum, as well as in U-937 cells[84].

As discussed, LTE_4 remains the least studied individual cys-LT. In addition to striking differences in reported activity of LTE_4 between tissues, there are observations suggesting a separate subclass of $CysLT_1$ receptor for LTE_4 in the guinea-pig trachea[83,85]. However, differences in the intrinsic agonist activity of LTE_4 compared with LTD_4 and LTE_4 could also contribute to these observations.

Another factor which may deserve attention is the localization of receptors to subcellular structures. The recent indications that LT biosynthesis occurs at the perinuclear membrane[86,87] raises the possibility that certain receptors may be localized in or close to the nucleus whereas others may be membrane associated. The observation that drugs which affect LT synthesis and receptors may interfere with the cellular transport of LTC_4[88] is also suggestive of a rather complicated inter-relationship between receptors, biosynthetic enzymes and transport mechanisms. It is tempting to speculate that there are as yet unknown relationships between receptors and transport mechanisms, biosynthetic enzymes and other proteins which may compete for the endogenous ligands.

The current classification is mainly derived from results in functional studies. There is supporting evidence from ligand-binding studies, in particular for the BLT receptor. However, binding studies designed to study cys-LTs have been more difficult to interpret, as discussed in detail in Chapter 4 of this volume. The signalling events following activation of LT receptors are also reviewed in Chapter 4.

In brief, although specific binding sites for LTD_4 have been identified in many tissues[89,90], including the human lung[91], radioligand binding studies with LTC_4 in lung and other tissues have often shown a less evident correlation between binding and functional responses[92–94]. It has been shown that LTC_4 also binds effectively to a liver glutathione S-transferase[95]. In view of the family of related enzymes with capacity to synthesize LTC_4[96], it appears that many enzymes and transport mechanisms[88] also display a high affinity for LTC_4 and the other cys-LTs. Increased knowledge of the cell biology of LT synthesis and transport may be required to resolve some of these problems, as well as the definition of the molecular structure and anchorage of LT receptors to subcellular constituents.

CONCLUSIONS

The $CysLT_1$ receptor antagonists are currently being introduced as a new therapy for asthma and perhaps, in the future, also as treatment for other inflammatory disorders. These achievements have been reached by the application of classical strategies such as the organic synthesis of new chemical entities, pharmacological screening in smooth muscle bioassays and subsequent clinical testing in healthy subjects and patients with asthma.

In parallel, the further exploration of LT effects and the application of currently available antagonists have established that there are certain actions of cys-LTs which are resistant to inhibition by the present class of antagonists. These include both contraction and relaxation of human pulmonary arteries and veins. This has led to the classification of such receptors as $CysLT_2$. There is no selective $CysLT_2$ antagonist available, but the structural analogue of cys-LTs BAY u9773 has been shown to competitively antagonize cys-LTs at both the $Cys\text{-}LT_1$ and the $CysLT_2$ receptor. Further subclasses of the $CysLT$ receptors are to be expected however on the basis of, for example, quite remarkable differences in sensitivity to agonists and antagonists between tissues, even in the same species. Although most effects of cys-LTs which may be involved in the pathogenesis of asthma are believed to be susceptible to $CysLT_1$-antagonism, a complete understanding of the role of cys-LTs in asthma will necessitate not only the molecular characterization of the receptors but also the development of selective agonists and antagonists at different receptor subclasses. This would also aid the definition of the role of cys-LTs in other pulmonary and extra-pulmonary diseases. For example, the potent cardiovascular effects of cys-LTs[60–63,97,98] suggest that it will be of great importance to assess which receptors are involved. Presumably in the future more selective antagonists will be required to provide precise and effective manipulation of LTs.

Acknowledgements

The author is supported by Karolinska Institutet and the following Swedish foundations: Medical Research Council (project 14X-9071), Heart Lung Foundation, the Foundation for Health Care Sciences and Allergy Research (Vårdal), and the Association Against Asthma and Allergy.

References

1. Borgeat P, Samuelsson B. Transformation of arachidonic acid by rabbit polymorphonuclear leukocytes. Formation of a novel dihydroxy eicosanoic acid. J Biol Chem. 1979; 254: 2643–6.
2. Borgeat P, Hamberg M, Samuelsson B. Transformation of arachidonic acid and homo-τ-linolenic acid by rabbit polymorphonuclear leukocytes. Monohydroxyacids from novel lipoxygenases. J Biol Chem 1976; 251: 7816–20 (Correction 1977; 252: 8772).
3. Hansson G, Lindgren JÅ, Dahlén S-E, Hedqvist P, Samuelsson B. Identification and biological activity of novel ω-oxidized metabolites of leukotriene B_4 from human leukocytes. FEBS Lett. 1981; 130: 107–12.
4. Piper PJ, Samhoun MN. Stimulation of arachidonic acid metabolism and generation of thromboxane A_2 by leukotrienes B_4, C_4 and D_4 in guinea-pig lung in vitro. Br J Pharmacol. 1982; 77: 267–75.
5. Sirois P, Roy S, Borgeat P, Picard S, Vallerand P. Evidence for a mediator role of thromboxane A_2 in the myotropic action of leukotriene B_4 (LTB_4) on the guinea-pig lung. Prostagl Leuko Med 1982; 8: 157–70.
6. Ford-Hutchinson AW, Bray MA, Doig MV, Shipley ME, Smith MJH. Leukotriene B_4, a potent chemokinetic and aggregating substance released from polymorphonuclear leukocytes. Nature. 1980; 286: 264–5.
7. Dahlén S-E, Björk J, Hedqvist P, Arfors K-E, Hammarström S, Lindgren JÅ, Samuelsson B. Leukotrienes promote plasma leakage and leukocyte adhesion in postcapillary venules: in vivo effects with relevance to the acute inflammatory response. Proc Natl Acad Sci USA. 1981; 78: 3887–91.
8. Bray MA, Ford-Hutchinson AW, Smith MJH. Leukotriene B_4: An inflammatory mediator in vivo. Prostaglandins. 1981; 22: 213–22.

9. Lindbom L, Hedqvist P, Dahlén S-E, Lindgren JÅ, Arfors KE. Leukotriene B_4 induces extravasation and migration of polymorphonuclear leukocytes in vivo. Acta Physiol Scand. 1982; 116: 105–8.

10. Smith MJH, Ford-Hutchinson AW, Bray MA. Leukotriene B: A potential mediator of inflammation. J Pharm Pharmacol. 1980; 32: 517–18.

11. Sehmi R, Wardlaw AJ, Cromwell O, Kurihawa K, Waltman P, Kay AB. Interleukin-5 selectively enhances the chemotactic response of eosinophils obtained from normal but not eosinophilic subjects. Blood. 1992; 79: 2952–9.

12. Yamaoka KA, Kolb JP. Leukotriene B_4 induces interleukin-5 generation from human T lymphocytes. Eur J Immunol 1993; 23: 2392–8.

13. Hafström I, Palmblad J, Malmsten C, Rådmark O, Samuelsson B. Leukotriene B_4-A stereospecific stimulator for release of lysosomal enzymes from neutrophils. FEBS Lett 1981; 130: 14–17.

14. Rae SA, Smith MJH. The stimulation of lysosomal enzyme secretion from human polymorphonuclear leukocytes by leukotriene B_4. J Pharm Pharmacol. 1981; 33: 616–18.

15. Claesson HE, Odlander B, Jakobsson PJ. Leukotriene B_4 in the immune system. Int J Immunopharmacol. 1982; 14: 441–9.

16. Yamaoka KA, Dugas B, Paul-Eugense N, Mencia-Huerta JM, Braquet P, Kolb JP. Leukotriene B_4 enhances IL-4 induced IgE production from normal human lymphocytes. Cell Immunol. 1994; 156: 124–34.

17. Devchand PR, Keller H, Peters JM, Vazques M, Gonzalez FJ, Wahli W. The $PPAR_\alpha$-leukotriene B_4 pathway to inflammation control. Nature. 1996; 384: 39–43.

18. Serhan CN. Signalling the fat controller. Nature. 1996; 384: 23–4.

19. Lewis RA, Goetzl EJ, Drazen JM, Soter NA, Austen KF, Corey EJ. Functional characterization of synthetic leukotriene B_4 and its stereochemical isomeres. J Exp Med. 1981; 154: 1243–8.

20. Strömberg F, Hamberg M, Rosenqvist U, Dahlén S-E, Haeggström JZ. Formation of a novel enzymatic metabolite of leukotriene A_4 in tissues of *Xenopus laevis*. Eur J Biochem. 1996; 238: 599–605.

21. Coleman RA, Eglen RM, Jones RL, et al. Prostanoid and Leukotriene Receptors: A Progress Report from the IUPHAR Working Parties on Classification and Nomenclature. Adv Prostag Thrombox Leukotriene Res. 1994; 23: 283–5.

22. Kreisle RA, Parker CW. Specific binding of leukotriene B_4 to a receptor on human polymorphonuclear leukocytes. J Exp Med. 1983; 157: 628–32.

23. Lin AH, Ruggsed PL, Gorman RR. Leukotriene B_4 binding to human neutrophils. Prostaglandins. 1984; 28: 837–45.

24. Goldman DW, Chang FH, Gifford LA, Goetzl EJ, Bourne HR. Pertussis toxin inhibition of chemotactic factor induced calcium mobilization and function in human polymorphonuclear leukocytes. J Exp Med. 1985; 162: 145–56.

25. Votta B, Mong S. Transition of affinity states for leukotriene B_4 receptor in sheep lung membranes. J Pharm Exp Ther. 1990; 265: 841–7.

26. Evans JF, Leblanc Y, Fitzsimmons BJ, Chorlesm S, Nathaniel D, Leveille C. Activation of leukocyte movements and displacement of ^{3}H-leukotriene B_4 from leukocyte membrane preparations by (12R)- and (12S)-hydroxyeicosatetraenoic acid. Biochem Biophys Acta. 1987; 917: 406–10.

27. Morris J. Wishka DG. Synthesis of novel antagonists of leukotriene B_4. Tetrahedron Lett. 1988; 29: 143–6.

28. Evans DJ, Barnes PJ, Spaethe SM, van Alstyne EL, Mitchell MI, O'Connor BJ. Effects of a leukotriene B_4 receptor antagonist, LY293111, on allergen-induced responses in asthma. Thorax. 1996; 51: 1178–84.

29. Yokomizo T, Izumi T, Chang K, Takuwa Y, Shimizu T. A G-protein-coupled receptor for leukotriene B4 that mediates chemotaxis. Nature. 1997; 387: 620–4.

30. Owman C, Nilsson C, Lolait SJ. Cloning of cDNA encoding a putative chemoattractant receptor. Genomics 1996; 37: 187–94.

31. Feinmark SJ, Lindgren JA, Claesson HE, Malmsten C, Samuelsson B. Stimulation of human leukocyte degranulation by leukotriene B_4 and its ω-oxidized metabolites. FEBS Lett. 1981; 136: 141–8.

32. Saad M, Wong K. Specific binding of leukotriene B_4 to guinea pig lung membranes. Biochem Biophys Res Commun. 1985; 143: 364–71.

33. Murphy RC, Hammarström S, Samuelsson B. Leukotriene C. A slow reacting substance from murine mastocytoma cells. Proc Natl Acad Sci USA. 1979; 76: 4275–9.

34. Morris HR, Taylor GW, Piper PJ, Tippins JR. Structure of slow-reacting substance of anaphylaxis from guinea-pig lung. Nature. 1980; 285: 104–6.

35. Parker CW, Falkenhein SF, Huber MM. Sequential conversion of the glutathionyl side chain of slow reacting substance (SRS) to cysteinyl-glycine and cysteine in rat basophilic leukemia cells stimulated with A 23187. Prostaglandins. 1980; 20: 863–86.

36. Örning L, Hammarström S, Samuelsson B. Leukotriene D. A slow reacting substance from rat basophilic leukemia cells. Proc Natl Acad Sci USA. 1980; 77: 2014–17.

37. Bach MK, Brashler JR, Brooks CD, Neerken AJ. Slow reacting substances: Comparison of some properties of human lung SRS-A and two distinct fractions from ionophore-induced rat mononuclear cells SRS. J Immunol. 1980; 122: 160–5.

38. Lewis RA, Austen KF, Drazen JM, Clark DA, Marfat A, Corey EJ. Slow reacting substances of anaphylaxis: Identification of leukotrienes C-1 and D from human and rat sources. Proc Natl Acad Sci USA. 1980; 77: 3710–14.

39. Sok DE, Pai JK, Atrache V, Sih CJ. Characterization of slow reacting substances (SRSs) of rat basophilic leukemia (RBL-1) cells. Effects of cysteine on SRS profile. Proc Natl Acad Sci USA. 1980; 77: 6481–5.

40. Bernström K, Hammarström S. Metabolism of leukotriene D by porcine kidney. J Biol Chem. 1981; 256: 9579–82.

41. Dahlén S-E, Hansson G, Hedqvist P, Björk T, Granström E, Dahlén B. Allergen challenge of lung tissue from asthmatics elicits bronchial contraction that correlates with the release of leukotrienes C_4, D_4 and E_4. Proc Natl Acad Sci USA. 1983; 80: 1712–16.

42. Orange RP, Austen KF. Slow reacting substance of anaphylaxis. Adv Immunol. 1969; 10: 105–44.

43. Drazen JM, Austen KF, Lewis RA, Clark DA, Goto G, Corey EJ. Comparative airway and vascular activities of leukotrienes C-1 and D in vivo and in vitro. Proc Natl Acad Sci USA. 1980; 77: 4354–8.

44. Hedqvist P, Dahlén S-E, Gustafsson LE, Hammarström S, Samuelsson B. Biological profile of leukotrienes C_4 and D_4. Acta Physiol Scand. 1980; 110: 331–3.

45. Dahlén S-E, Hedqvist P, Hammarström S, Samuelsson B. Leukotrienes are potent constrictors of human bronchi. Nature. 1980; 288: 484–6.

46. Hanna CJ, Bach MK, Pare PD, Schellenberg RR. Slow reacting substances (leukotrienes) contract human airway and pulmonary vascular smooth muscle. Nature. 1981; 290: 343–4.

47. Jones TR, Davies C, Daniel EE. Pharmacological study of the contractile activity of leukotriene C_4 and D_4 on isolated human airway smooth muscle. Can J Physiol Pharmacol. 1982; 60: 638–43.

48. Hau X-Y, Dahlén S-E, Lundberg JM, Hammarström S, Hedqvist P. Leukotrienes C_4, D_4 and E_4 cause extensive and widespread plasma extravasation in the guinea pig. Naunyn-Schmiedeberg's Arch Pharmacol. 1985; 330: 136–41.

49. Gardiner PJ, Abram TS, Cuthbert NJ. Evidence for two leukotriene receptor types in the guinea-pig isolated ileum. Eur J Pharmacol 1990; 182: 291–9.

50. Weichman BM, Muccitelli Rm, Osborn RR, Holden DA, Gleason JG, Wasserman MA. In vitro and in vivo mechanisms of leukotriene-mediated bronchoconstriction in the guinea pig. J Pharm Exp Ther. 1982; 222: 202–8.

51. Lee TH, Austen KF, Corey EJ, Drazen JM. LTE_4-induced airway hyperresponsiveness of guinea pig tracheal smooth muscle to histamine and evidence for three separate sulfidopeptide receptors. Proc Natl Acad Sci USA. 1984; 81: 4922–5.

52. Jacques CAJ, Spur BW, Johnson M, Lee TH. The mechanism of LTE_4-induced histamine hyperresponsiveness in guinea-pig tracheal and human bronchial smooth muscle in vitro. Br J Pharmacol. 1991; 104: 859–66.

53. Buckner CK, Fedyna JS, Robertson JL, Will JA, England DM, Krell RD, Saban R. Examination of the influence of the epithelium on contractile responses to peptidoleukotrienes and blockade by ICI 204, 219 in isolated guinea-pig trachea and human intralobar airways. J Pharm Exp Ther. 1990; 252: 77–85.

54. Buckner CK, Krell RD, Laravuso RB, Coursin DB, Bernstein PR, Will JA. Pharmacologic evidence that human intralobar airways do not contain different receptors that mediate contractions to leukotriene C_4 and D_4. J Pharm Exp Ther. 1986; 237: 558–62.

55. Samhoun MN, Conroy DM, Piper PJ. Pharmacological profile of leukotrienes E_4, N-acetyl-leukotriene E_4 and four of their novel omega- and beta-oxidative metabolites in airways of guinea-pig and man in vitro. Br J Pharmacol. 1989; 98: 1406–12.

56. Labat C, Ortiz JL, Norel X, et al. A second cysteinyl leukotriene receptor in human lung. J Pharm Exp Ther. 1992; 263: 800–5.

57. Coles SJ, Neill KH, Reid LM, et al. Effects of leukotrienes C_4 and D_4 on glycoprotein and lysozyme secretion by human bronchial mucosa. Prostaglandins. 1982; 25: 155–70.

58. Marom Z, Shelhamer JH, Bach MK, Morton DR, Kaliner M. Slow reacting substances, leukotrienes C_4 and D_4, increase the release of mucus from human airways in vitro. Am Rev Resp. Dis. 1982; 126: 449–51.

59. Peatfield AC, Piper PJ, Richardson PS. The effects of leukotriene C_4 on mucin release into the cat trachea in vivo and in vitro. Br J Pharmacol. 1982; 77: 391–3.

60. Terashita ZI, Fuki H, Hirata M, et al. Coronary vasoconstriction and PGI_2 release by leukotrienes in isolated guinea pig hearts. Eur J Pharmacol. 1981; 73: 357–61.

61. Letts LG, Piper PJ. The actions of leukotrienes C_4 and D_4 on guinea-pig isolated hearts. Br J Pharmacol. 1982; 76: 169–76.

62. Michelassi F, Landa L, Hill RD, Lowenstein E, Watkins WD, Petkau AJ, Zapol WM. Leukotriene D_4: A potent coronary artery vasoconstrictor associated with impaired ventricular contraction. Science. 1982; 217: 841–3.

63. Burke JA, Levi R, Guo Z-g, Corey EJ, Leukotrienes C_4, D_4 and E_4: Effects on human and guinea-pig cardiac preparations in vitro. J Pharm Exp Ther. 1982; 221: 235–41.

64. Laitinen L, Laitinen A, Haahtela T, Vilkka V, Spur B, Lee TH. Leukotriene E_4 causes granulocyte infiltration into asthmatic airways. Lancet. 1993; 341: 989–90.

65. Diamant Z, Hiltermann JT, van Rensen EL, et al. The effect of inhaled leukotriene D_4 and methacholine on sputum cell differentials in asthma. Am J Resp Crit Care Med. 1977; 155: 1247–53.

66. Underwood DC, Osborn RR, Newsholme SJ, Torphy TJ, Hay DWP. Persistent airway eosinophilia after leukotriene (LT) D_4 administration in the guinea-pig: Modulation by the LTD_4 receptor antagonist pranlukast or an interleukin-5 monoclonal antibody. Am J Resp Crit Care Med. 1996; 154: 850–7.

67. Munoz NM, Douglas I, Mayer I, Herrnreiter A, Zhu X, Leff AR. Eosinophil chemotaxis inhibited by 5-lipoxygenase blockade and leukotriene receptor antagonism. Am J Resp Crit Care Med. 1997; 155: 1398–403.

68. Peppelenbosch MP, Teretoolen LGJ, Hage WJ, de Laat SW. Epidermal growth factor-induced actin remodeling is regulated by 5-lipoxygenase and cyclooxygenase products. Cell. 1993; 74: 565–75.

69. Rajah R, Nunn SE, Herrick DJ, Grunstein MM, Cohen P. Leukotriene D_4 induces MMP-1, which functions as an IGFBP protease in human airway smooth muscle cells. Am J Physiol. 1996; 271: L1014–L1022.

70. Wang CG, Du T, Xu LJ, Martin JG. Role of leukotriene D_4 in allergen-induced increases in airway smooth muscle in the rat. Am Rev Resp Dis. 1993; 148: 413–17.

71. Augstein J, Farmer JB, Lee TB, Sheard P, Tattersall ML. Selective inhibitor of slow reacting substance of anaphylaxis. Nature New Biol. 1973; 245: 215–17.

72. Fleisch JH, Rinkema LE, Baker SR. Evidence for multiple leukotriene D_4 receptors in smooth muscle. Life Sci. 1982; 31: 577–81.

73. Krell RD, Tsai BS, Berdoulay A, Barone M, Giles RE. Heterogeneity of leukotriene receptors in the guinea-pig trachea. Prostaglandins. 1983; 25: 171–8.

74. Snyder DW, Krell RD. Pharmacologic evidence for a distinct leukotriene C_4 receptor in guinea-pig trachea. J Pharm Exp Ther. 1984; 231: 616–22.

75. Charette L, Jones TR. Effects of L-Serine borate on antagonism of leukotriene C_4-induced contractions of guinea-pig trachea. Br J Pharmacol. 1987; 91: 179–88.

76. Morris HR, Taylor GW, Jones CM, Piper PJ, Samhoun MN, Tippins JR. Slow-reacting substances (leukotrienes): Enzymes involved in their biosynthesis. Proc Natl Acad Sci USA. 1982; 79: 4838–42.

77. Yamaguchi T, Kohrogi H, Honda I, et al. A novel leukotriene antagonist, ONO-1078, inhibits and reverses human bronchial contraction induced by leukotrienes C_4 and D_4, and antigen in vitro. Am Rev Resp Dis. 1992; 146: 923–9.

78. Snyder DW, Krell RD. Pharmacology of peptide leukotrienes on ferret isolated airway smooth muscle. Prostaglandins. 1986; 32: 189–200.

79. Bäck M, Wikström-Jonsson E, Dahlén S-E. The cysteinyl-leukotriene antagonist BAY u9773 is a competitive antagonist of leukotriene C_4 in the guinea-pig ileum. Eur J Pharmacol. 1996; 317: 107–13.

80. Tudhope SR, Cuthbert NJ, Abram TS. et al. BAY u9773, a novel antagonist of cysteinyl-leukotrienes with activity against two receptor subtypes. Eur J Pharmacol. 1994; 264: 317–23.

81. Wilkström-Jonsson E. Functional characterisation of receptors for cysteinyl-leukotrienes in sheep trachealis muscle. Pulm Pharmacol Ther 1997; 10: 29–36.

82. Ortiz JL, Gorenne I, Cortijo J, et al. Leukotriene receptors on human pulmonary vascular endothelium. Br J Pharmacol. 1995; 115: 1382–6.

83. Aharony D, Catanese CA, Falcone RC. Kinetic and pharmacologic analysis of [^{3}H] leukotriene E_4 binding to receptors on guinea pig lung membranes: Evidence for selective binding to a subset of leukotriene D_4 receptors. J Pharm Exp Ther. 1989; 248: 581–8.

84. Wetmore LA, Gerard NP, Herron DK, et al. Leukotriene receptors on U-937 cells: II discriminatory responses to leukotrienes C_4 and D_4. Am J Physiol. 1991; 261: L164–L171.

85. Hay DWP, Muccitelli RM, Wilson KA, Wasserman MA, Torphy TJ. Functional antagonism by salbutamol suggests differences in the relative efficacies and dissociation constants of the peptidoleukotrienes in guinea-pig trachea. J Pharm Exp Ther. 1987; 244: 71–8.

86. Woods JW, Evans JF, Ethier D. 5-Lipoxygenase and 5-lipoxygenase activating protein are localized in the nuclear envelope of activated human leukocytes. J. Exp Med. 1993; 178: 1935–46.

87. Peters-Golden M, McNish R. Redistribution of 5-lipoxygenase and cytosolic phospholipase A_2 to the nuclear fraction upon macrophage activation. Biochem Biophys Res Commun. 1993; 196: 147–53.

88. Leier I, Jedlitschky G, Buchholz U, Cole SPC, Deeley RG, Keppler D. The MRP gene encodes an ATP-dependent export pump for leukotriene C_4 and structurally related conjugates. J Biol Chem. 1994; 269: 27807–10.

89. Bruns REF, Thomsen WJ, Pugsley TA. Binding of leukotrienes C_4 and D_4 to membranes from guinea-pig lung: regulation by ions and guanine nucleotides. Lif Sci. 1983; 33: 645–53.

90. Pong SS, DeHaven R. Characterisation of a leukotriene D_4 receptor in guinea pig lung. Proc Natl Acad Sci USA. 1983; 80: 7415–20.

91. Lewis MA, Mong S, Vaseella RL, Crooke ST. Characterization of leukotriene D_4 receptors in adult and fetal human lung. Biochem Pharmacol. 1985; 34: 4311–17.

92. Nicosia S, Crowley HJ, Olivia D, Welton AF. Binding sites for ^{3}H-LTC$_4$ in membranes from guinea pig ileal longitudinal muscle. Prostaglandins. 1984; 27: 483–94.

93. Rovati GE, Olivia D, Sautebin L, Folco GC, Welton AF, Nicosia S. Identification of specific binding sites for leukotriene C_4 in membranes from human lung. Biochem Pharmacol. 1985; 34: 2831–7.

94. Civelli M, Olivia D, Mezzetti M, Nicosia S. Characteristics and distribution of specific binding sites for leukotriene C_4 in human bronchi. J Pharmacol Exp Ther. 1987; 242: 189–98.

95. Sun FF, Chau L-Y, Spur B, Corey EJ, Lewis RA, Austen KF. Identification of a high affinity leukotriene C_4-binding protein in rat liver cytosol as glutathione S-transferase. J Biol Chem. 1986; 261: 8540–6.

96. Jakobsson PJ, Mancini JA, Ford-Hutchinson AW. Identification and characterisation of a novel human microsomal gluthathione S-transferase with leukotriene C_4 synthase activity and significant sequence identity to 5-lipoxygenase activating protein and leukotriene C_4 synthase. J Biol Chem. 1996; 271: 22203–10.

97. Smedegård G, Hedqvist P, Dahlén S-E, Revenäs B, Hammarström S, Samuelsson B. Leukotriene C_4 affects pulmonary and cardiovascular dynamics in the monkey. Nature. 1982; 295: 327–9.

98. Sala A, Rossoni G, Buccellati C, Berti F, Folco G, Maclouf J. Formation of sulphidopeptide-leukotrienes by cell-cell interaction causes coronary vasoconstriction in isolated, cell-perfused heart of rabbit. Br J Pharmacol. 1993; 110: 1206–12.
99. Dahlén S-E, Serhan CN. Lipoxins: Bioactive lipoxygenase interaction products. In: Crooke ST, Wong A, editors. Lipoxygenases and Their Products. San Diego: Academic Press, 1992: 235–75.

3 Enzymes involved in the production of leukotrienes and related molecules

A. W. FORD-HUTCHINSON and P.-J. JAKOBSSON

Leukotriene (LT) receptor activation (*CysLT* and BLT) has been postulated to be involved in the induction of inflammatory and immediate hypersensitivity responses[1-3]. In particular, LTs have been implicated in the pathology of human bronchial asthma[4], and two *CysLT$_1$* receptor antagonists (montelukast and zafirlukast) and one 5-lipoxygenase (5-LO) inhibitor (zileuton) have been approved for the treatment of human bronchial asthma in several countries outside Japan. In theory LT biosynthesis inhibitors might have advantages over *CysLT$_1$* receptor antagonists as LTB$_4$ has been suggested to be a mediator of inflammatory conditions[3]. However, there is no evidence that such inhibitors have advantages in the treatment of human bronchial asthma. In particular, a BLT receptor antagonist has been shown to inhibit neutrophil accumulation following antigen challenge of asthmatic subjects with no effect on clinical parameters, arguing against a role for either BLT receptor activation or neutrophil accumulation in this disease[5]. With regard to other inflammatory diseases, in psoriasis there is no evidence in clinical trials that LT biosynthesis inhibitors have any clinical efficacy and this has been used to argue that 5-LO activation has no role in this disease[6]. Another disease in which LTB$_4$ has been postulated to be a mediator is inflammatory bowel disease[7]. However, a double blind clinical trial has been carried out in patients with ulcerative colitis using doses of the LT biosynthesis inhibitor MK-591 that produced a 100% inhibition of LT biosynthesis over a 24 h period as measured in various assays[8]. In this trial, MK-591 produced effects that were no different to current therapy (sulphasalazine), suggesting that LTs do not have a major role in the pathology of this disease. Whether LTs have a role in other inflammatory diseases, such as glomerulonephritis, remains to be fully explored.

Leukotrienes are synthesized from arachidonic acid through the action of 5-LO in concert with its activating protein, 5-LO activating protein (FLAP). This chapter briefly describes the properties of 5-LO and concentrates on the description of a family of proteins that includes FLAP, LTC$_4$ synthase and a series of related proteins with glutathione S-transferase and glutathione peroxidase activities.

5-LIPOXYGENASE

5-Lipoxygenase is a member of a group of lipoxygenase enzymes that include 12- and 15-lipoxygenases. These enzymes catalyse the addition of molecular oxygen to a 1,4-*cis, cis*-pentadiene moiety to produce a 1-hydroperoxy-2,4-*trans, cis*-pentadiene unit[9].

Following cellular activation 5-LO is activated by a rise in intracellular calcium. This activation causes the enzyme to translocate from either the cytosol or within the nucleus (depending upon the cell type) to the nuclear envelope[10,11]. It has been suggested that the role of calcium is to cause the enzyme to attach itself to phospholipid membranes in a way similar to that reported for protein kinase-C, cytosolic phospholipase A_2 and other calcium-dependent enzymes whose substrates are found either in micelles, membranes or other aggregated structures[12]. In addition to stimulation by calcium, 5-LO activity is also reported to be stimulated by ATP and inhibited by guanine nucleotides. The enzyme contains a non-haem arm coordinated to the carboxyl terminal and two of five clustered histidine residues which are highly conserved in all lipoxygenase sequences known to date[13]. This non-haem iron catalyses the redox reactions associated with arachidonic oxygenation. Because of the redox nature of the enzyme, a number of compounds can act as reducing agents for the enzyme by participating as substrates for a pseudoperoxidase activity of the enzyme[14]. Such compounds are considered 5-LO inhibitors but in general have not proven particularly useful as drug candidates. Competitive inhibitors of 5-LO, including the thiopyranoindole inhibitors described by Merck Frosst[15] and the methoxyalkyl thiazole class of inhibitors described by Zeneca[16], have also been described.

5-LIPOXYGENASE ACTIVATING PROTEIN (FLAP)

The discovery of FLAP came about through the elucidation of the mechanism of action of LT biosynthesis inhibitors such as MK-886 (3[1-(4-chlorobenzyl-3-*t*-butyl-thio-5-isopropyl-2-yl)-2,2-dimethyl-propanoic acid]) and related compounds[17,18]. Such compounds were found to be potent inhibitors of leukotriene biosynthesis in intact cells but had no effect upon either the 5-LO enzyme or on the availability of substrate. Initial studies indicated that these compounds inhibited an activation step for 5-LO as evidenced by a concentration-dependent inhibition of 5-LO translocation to a membrane site from the cytosol[18]. In order to define a molecular target for MK-886, radioactive photoaffinity probes were synthesized and shown to bind in a competable manner to an 18 kDa internal membrane protein present only in cells with LT biosynthetic capacity[19]. This protein was isolated and purified from solubilized membranes through the aid of affinity columns to which MK-886 had been coupled, the 18 kDa protein was then sequenced and sequence data was used to obtain the rat cDNA and in turn the human cDNA[19,20]. Dual transfection experiments were then used to show that this 18 kDa protein was necessary for cellular LT biosynthesis and it was termed 5-lipoxygenase activating protein (FLAP)[20].

It was originally suggested that FLAP would act as a 'docking' protein for 5-LO following its translocation from the cytosol to a membrane site. This would require the formation of a stable complex at the membrane between activated 5-LO, FLAP as well as possibly other components of the LT biosynthetic machinery, such as cytosolic phospholipase A_2. However, a number of studies has shown a lack of correlation between inhibition of translocation and inhibition of LT biosynthesis[21–24]. Current evidence, based in part on the use of a novel photoaffinity analogue of arachidonic acid, has suggested that FLAP may act as a fatty acid transfer protein for arachidonic acid facilitating the transfer of arachidonic acid to 5-LO[25]. This allows for the enzymic reaction to occur in a more efficient way resulting in an increased synthesis of LTA_4 as opposed to 5-hydroperoxyeicosatetraenoic acid[26,27].

Immunoelectron microscopic labelling of ultrathin frozen sections has been used to study the subcellular localization of FLAP and other components of the LT biosynthetic pathway[11,28]. These studies have demonstrated that FLAP is localized to the lumen of the nuclear envelope and the associated endoplasmic reticulum. In resting cells 5-LO is present either in the cytosol or the nucleus depending on the cell type. Following cellular activation, 5-LO can then be found, together with cytosolic phospholipase A_2, at the same site as FLAP. The biological significance of intranuclear 5-LO in certain cells is unclear. The proposed mechanism for LT biosynthesis in intact cells is shown in Figure 1 together with the mechanisms of inhibition of LT biosynthesis by FLAP inhibitors such as MK-886.

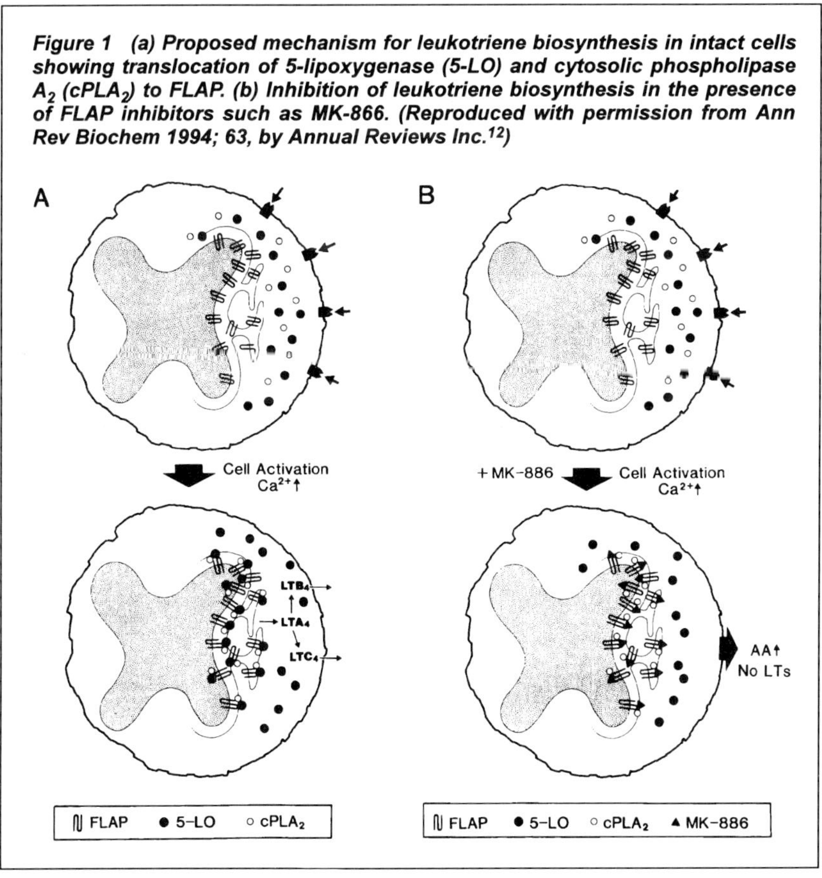

Figure 1 *(a) Proposed mechanism for leukotriene biosynthesis in intact cells showing translocation of 5-lipoxygenase (5-LO) and cytosolic phospholipase A_2 (cPLA₂) to FLAP. (b) Inhibition of leukotriene biosynthesis in the presence of FLAP inhibitors such as MK-866. (Reproduced with permission from Ann Rev Biochem 1994; 63, by Annual Reviews Inc.[12])*

MICROSOMAL GLUTATHIONE S-TRANSFERASE I

Microsomal glutathione S-transferase I (MGST-I) was isolated in 1982[29]. This 17 kDa enzyme has a wide substrate specificity and is predominantly expressed in liver microsomes. Substrates for this enzyme are halogenated arenes, typified by 1-chloro-2,4-dinitrobenzene, as well as various polyhalogenated unsaturated hydrocarbons[30]. In contrast to certain cytosolic glutathione S-transferases, LTA_4 and other epoxides are poor substrates for MGST-I[31,32]. This enzyme should not, therefore, contribute to LTC_4 biosynthesis. In addition to the glutathione S-transferase activity, MGST-I also catalyses a glutathione-dependent reduction of certain lipid hydroperoxides such as organic hydroperoxides, fatty acid hydroperoxides and phospholipid hydroperoxides[33,34]. These reactions may be of importance for protection against membrane lipid peroxidation under conditions of oxidative stress[35]. A miscellaneous feature of MGST-I is the effective binding of LTC_4[36]. The role of this LTC_4 binding is not known and requires further studies but may suggest a storage function of the enzyme. MGST-I is active as a homotrimer, in contrast to LTC_4 synthase and the different cytosolic glutathione S-transferases which are active as dimers.

LTC_4 SYNTHASE

The cysteinyl leukotrienes (LTC_4, LTD_4 and LTE_4) are important mediators of airway obstruction. LTC_4 synthase specifically catalyses the conjugation of leukotriene A_4 with glutathione. LTC_4 synthase was successfully purified from THP-1 cells as an 18 kDa membrane associated protein, active as a homodimer[37]. Thereafter, two groups independently cloned and characterized the gene product[38,39]. The deduced amino acid sequence demonstrated that FLAP and LTC_4 synthase were members of the same gene family (31% identity). The LTC_4 synthase polypeptide also displayed a very similar hydropathy pattern to that of FLAP. The genes coding for FLAP and LTC_4 synthase are different in size but have the same intron/exon organization, consisting of five small exons and four large introns[40,41]. In a recent study, where several site directed mutants of LTC_4 synthase were investigated, it was concluded that Arg-51 functions as a proton donor for the opening of the LTA_4 epoxide and Tyr-93 as a base for the formation of the thiolate anion of glutathione[42].

DISCOVERY AND CHARACTERIZATION OF MICROSOMAL GLUTATHIONE S-TRANSFERASES II AND III

In order to investigate whether or not the FLAP/LTC_4 synthase gene family includes other members, the GenBank data base was searched for sequences homologous to FLAP and LTC_4 synthase. Recently, we reported on the characterization of MGST-II[43], an enzyme which catalyses both the formation of LTC_4 from LTA_4 and glutathione and the conjugation of glutathione with 1-chloro-2,4-dinitrobenzene (a common substrate for the majority of glutathione S-transferases). The apparent K_m for LTA_4 was 5 to 6 fold higher than that obtained with LTC_4 synthase. In addition to LTC_4 production, MGST-II also catalysed the formation of a LTC_4 isomer from LTA_4

and glutathione. This indicates less catalytic stereospecificity than LTC$_4$ synthase[44]. Based on these activities MGST-II forms an interesting link between MGST-I and LTC$_4$ synthase. Its biological function has to be further investigated. MGST-II protein expression was determined by Western blot and found predominantly in human liver microsomes and endothelial cells, and more sparsely in lung membranes[45].

Using the predicted amino acid sequence for MGST-II, the GenBank data base was again searched for related gene products. This revealed an expressed sequence tag (EST) clone with significant sequence identity with MGST-II, FLAP and LTC$_4$ synthase[46]. This novel protein was expressed in a baculovirus/insect cell system and such cells (*Spodoptera frugiperda*, Sf9) infected with recombinant baculovirus were tested for both LTC$_4$ synthase activity and the capacity to conjugate 1-chloro-2,4-dinitrobenzene with reduced glutathione. The capacity to produce LTC$_4$ was about one-third of the activity obtained in microsomes isolated from Sf9 cells infected with MGST-II. No glutathione S-transferase activity was found using 1-chloro-2,4-dinitrobenzene as substrate. Since MGST-I has been shown to function as a glutathione-dependent peroxidase towards various phospholipid and fatty acid hydroperoxides, this activity was investigated using 5(*S*)-hydroperoxy-8,11,14-*cis*-6-*trans*-eicosatetraenoic acid (5-HPETE) as substrate. Both MGST-II and the novel enzyme catalysed a glutathione-dependent reduction of 5-HPETE to 5-HETE. The apparent K_m for 5-HPETE was 7 µM for MGST-II and 21 µM for the novel enzyme. Based on these catalytic activities it was proposed that the novel microsomal enzyme was part of the glutathione S-transferase gene super family and was denoted microsomal glutathione S-transferase-III (MGST-III). The predicted amino acid sequence shows 36% identity to MGST-II (Figure 2). In agreement with data

---

Figure 2   Alignment of LTC$_4$ synthase, MGST-II and MGST-III. Conserved residues are shown in boldface type

```
                 1                                                          60

LTC₄ synthase    ~~~MkdEvaL LAAVtlLgvl lQAYFsLQVi sARrafrVsP Plt.TGpPE. ...FERVyRA

MGST-II          ~~~MagnsiL LAAVsiLSac qQsYFALQVg KARlKYKVtP Pav.TGsPE. ...FERVfRA

MGST-III         mavlskEygf vlltgaaSfi mvAhlAinVs KARkKYKVey PimystdPEn ghiFnciqRA


                 61                                                         120

LTC₄ synthase    QvNCsEyfPl FLaTLWVAGi fFHegaAalc GLVYlfaRlr YFqGYarsAq lRlaplyaSa

MGST-II          QQNCvEfYPi FiiTLWmAGw YFnqvfAtcL GLVYIyGRhL YFwGYseaAk kRitgfRlSL

MGST-III         hQNtlEvYPp FLffLaVgGv Y.HpriAsgL GLawIvGRvL YayGYytgep skrs..RgaL


                 121                                  159

LTC₄ synthase    raLwLLvaLa ALGllAhFLp aaLraaLlgr LRtllpwa

MGST-II          GiLALLtLLG ALGiansFLd eyLdlniakk LRrqf

MGST-III         GsiALLgLvG ttvcsAfqhl gwvksgLgsg pkcch
```

demonstrating that Arg-51 and Tyr-93 are crucial for LTC$_4$ synthase activity[42], corresponding amino acid residues are also found in both MGST-II and MGST-III (underlined in Figure 2). MGST-III also displays a similar hydropathy pattern to FLAP, LTC$_4$ synthase, MGST-I and MGST-II. Table 1 summarizes some basic parameters of the gene family. They are all of the same size, ranging from 147 to 161 amino acids. Only FLAP differs in its isoelectric point being more neutral than the other more basic members. They all reside on different chromosomes. Based on sequence comparisons, MGST-II is most related to LTC$_4$ synthase while MGST-III seems to be closest to MGST-II.

The expression of MGST-III mRNA was analysed by Northern blot. Table 2 summarizes the tissue distribution of MGST-II, MGST-III and FLAP. Both MGST-II and MGST-III are expressed in heart, skeletal muscle, adrenals and testis. In the liver and bone marrow they are expressed differently: MGST-I is heavily expressed in the liver, but also in organs such as adrenal, lung, intestine, spleen and heart[47,48]. In contrast, FLAP expression was restricted to cells and tissues expected to possess 5-LO, i.e. tissues with a high content of leukocytes such as peripheral blood leukocytes, bone marrow, spleen and lung.

CONCLUSIONS

A new gene family has been identified which includes a number of members with glutathione S-transferase activity as well as one protein, FLAP, without apparent enzymic activity. Proteins such as LTC$_4$ synthase appear to be specific for a single substrate, LTA$_4$. Others such as MGST-II and MGST-III possess both LTC$_4$ synthase activity as well as the capacity to reduce 5-HPETE to 5-HETE in the presence of reduced glutathione. With regard to these proteins, their biological activities require further investigation in order to clarify their biological significance. At this time we can only speculate upon their functions. Are they membrane associated equivalents of the various cytosolic glutathione S-transferases? If so, they would be part of the cellular defence system against toxic agents such as various xenobiotics, fatty acid expoxides, possibly derived from the cytochrome P$_{450}$ systems, and lipid hydroperoxides formed under conditions of oxidative stress. Alternatively, they may play a more specific role in defined metabolic pathways. For instance, prostaglandin (PG) H$_2$ can be enzymatically converted into either one of PGF$_{2\alpha}$, PGE$_2$ and PGD$_2$.

Table 1 Properties of the gene family consisting of MGST-I, FLAP, LTC$_4$ synthase, MGST-II and III

Protein	Amino acids	pI	Chromosome	% identity with MGST-II	% identity with MGST-III
FLAP	161	8.7	13q12	33	20
LTC$_4$ synthase	150	11.1	5q35	44	27
MGST-I	155	10.2	12	11	22
MGST-II	147	10.4	4q28–31	–	36
MGST-III	152	10.2	1q23	36	–

Table 2 Tissue distribution of MGST-II, MGST-III and FLAP by Northern blot analysis

Tissue	MGST-II	MGST-III	FLAP
Heart	+	++	-
Brain	-	+/-	-
Placenta	-	+	-
Lung	-	-	+
Liver	+	+/-	-
Spleen	+	+/-	+
Skeletal muscle	+	++	-
Pancreas	+/-	+/-	-
Adrenals	+++	+++	-
Testis	+	+	-
PBL	-	+/-	++
Bone marrow	-	+	++
HL60	+	-	+
HELA	+	+	-
KML	+	+	-
adenocarcinoma	+	+	-
lung carcinoma	-	+	-
melanoma	+/-	+	-
Raji	-	-	++
Molt4	-	-	+/-

The enzymes responsible for these conversions are not well characterized. However, PGE_2 synthase has been reported as a membrane-bound, 17 kDa, glutathione-dependent protein[49,50]. In addition, a novel $PGF_{2\alpha}$ synthase isolated from sheep seminal vesicles was recently reported as a membrane-associated 16.5 kDa, glutathione-dependent enzyme[51]. This protein also catalyses the reduction of an organic lipid hydroperoxide (cumene hydroperoxide). However, 1-chloro-2,4-dinitrobenzene was not a substrate for this enzyme. Therefore, this protein resembles MGST-III and may be a member of this gene family

References

1. Ford-Hutchinson AW. Leukotriene antagonists and inhibitors as modulators of IgE-mediated reactions. Springer Semin Immunopathol. 1993; 15: 37–50.
2. Piper PJ. Formation and actions of leukotrienes. Physiol Rev. 1984; 64: 744–61.
3. Ford-Hutchinson AW. Leukotriene B4 in inflammation. Crit Rev Immunol. 1990; 10: 1–12.
4. Pauwels RA, Joos GF, Kips JC. Leukotrienes as therapeutic target in asthma. Allergy. 1995; 50: 615–22.
5. Evans DJ, Barnes PJ, Spaethe SM, van Alstyne EL, Mitchell MI, O'Connor BJ. Effect of a leukotriene B_4 receptor antagonist, LY293111, on allergen induced responses in asthma. Thorax. 1996; 51: 1178–84.
6. Ford-Hutchinson AW. 5-Lipoxygenase activation in psoriasis; a dead issue? Skin Pharmacol. 1993; 6: 292–7.
7. Sharon P, Stenson WF. Enhanced synthesis of leukotriene B_4 by colonic mucosa in inflammatory bowel disease. Gastroenterology. 1984; 86: 453–60.
8. Roberts WG, Simon TJ, Berlin RG, et al. Leukotrienes in ulcerative colitis: results of a multicenter trial of a leukotriene biosynthesis inhibitor, MK-591. Gastroenterology. 1997: 112: 725–32.

9. Yamamoto S. Mammalian lipoxygenases: Molecular structures and functions. Biochim Biophys Acta. 1992; 1128: 117–31.

10. Rouzer CA, Kargman S. Translocation of 5-lipoxygenase to the membrane in human leukocytes challenged with ionophore A23187. J Biol Chem. 1988; 263: 10980–8.

11. Woods JW, Coffey MJ, Brock TG, Singer II, Peters-Golden M. 5-Lipoxygenase is located in the euchromatin of the nucleus in resting human alveolar macrophages and translocates to the nuclear envelope upon cell activation. J Clin Invest. 1995; 95: 2035–46.

12. Ford-Hutchinson AW, Gresser M, Young RN. 5-Lipoxygenase. Annu Rev Biochem. 1994; 63: 383–417.

13. Hammarberg T, Zhang Y-Y, Lind B, Radmark O, Samuelsson B. Mutations of the C-terminal isoleucine and other potential iron ligands of 5-lipoxygenase. Eur J Biochem. 1995; 230: 401–7.

14. Riendeau D, Falgueyret J-P, Guay J, Ueda N, Yamamoto S. Pseudoperoxidase activity of 5-lipoxygenase stimulated by potent benzofuranol and N-hydroxyurea inhibitors of the lipoxygenase reaction. Biochem J. 1991; 274: 287–92.

15. Hutchinson JH, Prasit P, Choo LY, et al. Development of L-689,065, the prototype of a new class of potent 5-lipoxygenase inhibitors. Bioorg Med Chem Lett. 1992; 2: 1699–702.

16. Bird TGC, Bruneau P, Crawley GC, et al. (Methoxyalkyl)thiazoles: a new series of potent, selective, and orally active 5-lipoxygenase inhibitors displaying high enantioselectivity. J Med Chem. 1991; 34: 2176–86.

17. Gillard J, Ford-Hutchinson AW, Chan C, et al. L-663–536 (Mk-886) (30[1-(4-chlorobenzyl)-3-*t*-butyl-thio-5-isopropylindol-2-yl]-2,2-dimethylpropanoic acid), a novel, orally active leukotriene biosynthesis inhibitor. Can J Physiol Pharmacol. 1989; 67: 456–64.

18. Rouzer CA, Ford-Hutchinson AW, Morton HE, Gillard JW. MK-886, a potent and specific leukotriene biosynthesis inhibitor blocks and reverses the membrane association of 5-lipoxygenase in ionophore-challenged leukocytes. J Biol Chem. 1990; 265: 1436–42.

19. Miller DK, Gillard JW, Vickers PJ, et al. Identification and isolation of a membrane protein necessary for leukotriene production. Nature. 1990; 343: 278–81.

20. Dixon RA, Diehl RE, Opas E, et al. Requirement of a 5-lipoxygenase-activating protein for leukotriene synthesis. Nature. 1990; 343: 282–4.

21. Coffey M, Peters-Golden M, Fantone JC III, Sporn PHS. Membrane association of active-5 lipoxygenase in resting cells. Evidence for novel regulation of the enzyme in the rat alveolar macrophage. J Biol Chem. 1992; 267: 570–6.

22. Kargman S, Vickers PJ, Evans JF. A23187-induced translocation of 5-lipoxygenase in osteosarcoma cells. J Cell Biol. 1992; 119: 1701–9.

23. Hatzelmann A, Fruchtmann R, Mohrs KH, Raddatz S, Muller-Peddinghaus R. Mode of action of the new selective leukotriene synthesis inhibitor BAY X 1005 ((*R*)-2[4-[quinolin-2-yl-methoxy]phenyl]2-cyclopentyl acetic acid) and structurally related compounds. Biochem Pharmacol. 1993; 45: 101–11.

24. Hatzelmann A, Fruchtmann R, Mohrs KH, et al. Mode of action of the leukotriene synthesis (FLAP) inhibitor BAY X1005. Implications for biological regulation of 5-lipoxygenase. Adv Prostaglandin Thrombox Leukot Res. 1994; 22: 23–31.

25. Mancini JA, Abromovitz M, Cox ME, et al. 5-Lipoxygenase-activating protein is an arachidonate binding protein. FEBS Lett. 1993; 318: 277–81.

26. Hill, E, Maclouf J, Murphy RC, Henson PM. Reversible membrane association of neutrophil 5-lipoxygenase is accompanied by retention of activity and a change in substrate specificity. J Biol Chem. 1992; 267: 22048–53.

27. Abramovitz M, Wong E, Cox ME, Richardson CD, Li C, Vickers PJ. 5-lipoxygenase activating protein stimulates the utilization of arachidonic acid by 5-lipoxygenase. Eur J Biochem. 1993; 215: 105–11.

28. Woods JW, Evans JF, Ethier D, et al. 5-lipoxygenase and 5-lipoxygenase-activating protein are localized in the nuclear envelope of activated human leukocytes. J Exp Med. 1993; 178: 1935–46.

29. Morgenstern R, Guthenberg C, Depierre JW. Microsomal glutathione S-transferase EC-2.5.1.18. Purification, initial characterization and demonstration that it is not identical to the cytosolic glutathione S-transferases A B and C. Eur J Biochem. 1982; 128: 243–8.

30. Andersson C, Mosialou E, Weinander R, Morgenstern R. Enzymology of microsomal glutathione S-transferase. Adv Pharmacol. 1994; 27: 19–35.

31. Morgenstern R, Lundqvist G, Hancock V, DePierre W. Studies on the activity and activation of rat liver microsomal glutathione transferase in particular with a substrate analogue series. J Biol Chem. 1988; 263: 6671–5.

32. Soderstrom M, Hammarström S, Mannervik B. Leukotriene C synthase in mouse mastocytoma cells, an enzyme distinct from cytosolic and microsomal glutathione transferases. Biochem J. 1988; 250: 713–18.

33. Morgenstern R, DePierre JW. Microsomal glutathione transferase. EC-2.5.1.18 purification in unactivated form and further characterization of the activation process, substrate specificity and amino acid composition. Eur J Biochem. 1983; 134: 591–8.

34. Mosialou E, Piemonte F, Andersson C, Vos R, van Bladeren P, Morgenstern R. Microsomal glutathione transferase lipid-derived substrates and lipid dependence. Arch Biochem Biophys. 1995; 320: 210–16.

35. Mosialou E, Ekstrom G, Adang AE, Morgenstern R. Evidence that rat liver microsomal glutathione transferase is responsible for glutathione-dependent protection against lipid peroxidation. Biochem Pharmacol. 1993; 45: 1645–51.

36. Metters KM, Sawyer N, Nicholson DW. Microsomal glutathione S-transferase is the predominant leukotriene C_4 binding site in cellular membranes. J Biol Chem. 1994; 269: 12816–23.

37. Nicholson DW, Ali A, Vaillancourt JP, et al. Purification to homogeneity and the N-terminal sequence of human leukotriene C_4 synthase: a homodimeric glutathione S-transferase composed of 18-kDa subunits. Proc Natl Acad Sci USA. 1993; 90: 2015–19.

38. Lam BK, Penrose JF, Freeman GJ, Austen KF. Expression cloning of a cDNA for human leukotriene C_4 synthase, an integral membrane protein conjugating reduced glutathione to leukotriene A_4. Proc Natl Acad Sci USA. 1994; 91: 7663–7.

39. Welsch DJ, Creely DP, Hauser SD, Mathis KJ, Krivi GG, Isakson PC. Molecular cloning and expression of human leukotriene C_4 synthase. Proc Natl Acad Sci USA. 1994; 91: 9745–9.

40. Kennedy BP, Diehl RE, Boie Y, Adam M, Dixon RA. Gene characterization and promoter analysis of the human 5-lipoxygenase-activating protein (FLAP). J Biol Chem. 1991; 266: 8511–16.

41. Penrose JF, Spector J, Baldasaro M, et al. Molecular cloning of the gene for human leukotriene C_4 synthase. J Biol Chem. 1996; 271: 11356–61.

42. Lam BK, Penrose JF, Xu K, Baldasaro MH, Austen KF. Site-directed mutagenesis of human leukotriene C_4 synthase. J Biol Chem. 1997; 272: 13923–8.

43. Jakobsson PJ, Mancini JA, Ford-Hutchinson AW. Identification and characterization of a novel human microsomal glutathione S-transferase with leukotriene C_4 synthase activity and significant sequence identity to 5-lipoxygenase activating protein and leukotriene C_4 synthase. J Biol Chem. 1996; 271: 22203–10.

44. Jakobsson PJ, Scoggan KA, Yergey J, Mancini J, Ford-Hutchinson AW. Characterization of a novel 17 kDa microsomal glutathione S-transferase by western blot and identification of a new metabolite of LTA_4 by mass spectrometry. J Lipid Mediat. 1997; 17: 15–20.

45. Scoggan K, Jakobsson PJ, Ford-Hutchinson AW. Production of leukotriene C_4 in different human tissues is attributable to distinct membrane bound biosynthetic enzymes. J Biol Chem. 1997; 272: 10182–7.

46. Jakobsson PJ, Mancini JA, Riendeau D, Ford-Hutchinson AW. Identification and characterization of a novel microsomal enzyme with glutathione-type dependent transferase and peroxidase activities. J Biol Chem. 1997; 272: 22934–9.

47. Dejong JL, Morgenstern R, Jornvall H, DePierre JW, Tu C-PD. Gene expression of rat and human microsomal glutathione S-transferases. J Biol Chem. 1988; 263: 8430–6.

48. Morgenstern R, Lundqvist G, Andersson G, Balk L, DePierre JW. The distribution of microsomal glutathione transferase among different organelles, different organs and different organisms. Biochem Pharmacol. 1984; 33: 3609–14.

49. Nugteren DH, Christ-Hazelhof E. Chemical and enzymic conversion of the prostaglandin endoperoxide PGH_2. Adv Prostaglandin Thromboxane Res. 1980; 6: 129–37.

50. Tanaka Y, Ward SL, Smith WL. Immunochemical and kinetic evidence for two different

prostaglandin H-prostaglandin E isomerases in sheep vesicular gland microsomes. J Biol Chem. 1987; 262: 1374–81.

51. Burgess JR, Reddy CC. Isolation and characterization of an enzyme from sheep seminal vesicles that catalyzes the glutathione-dependent reduction of prostaglandin H_2 to prostaglandin $F_{2\alpha}$. Biochem Mol Biol Int. 1997; 41: 217–26.

4 Cysteinyl-leukotriene receptors and transduction mechanisms in airway cells

S. NICOSIA, G. E. ROVATI, V. CAPRA, S. RAVASI,
M. MEZZETTI, T. VIGANÒ, M. R. ACCOMAZZO,
A. HERNANDEZ, A. BONAZZI, M. BOLLA, E. GALBIATI,
M. DI LUCA, A. CAPUTI, A. M. VILLA, S. ESPOSITO,
S. DOGLIA, M. ROVELLI and G. FOLCO

A variety of inflammatory cells synthesize cys-leukotrienes (cys-LTs) C_4, D_4 and E_4 in response to biological and non-biological stimuli[1]: eosinophils, basophils and mast cells[2,3] are able to synthesize cys-LTs from arachidonic acid but cys-LTs can also be produced through transcellular metabolism from neutrophil-derived LTA_4 by vascular endothelial cells[4-6] and platelets[7].

Cys-LTs are potent smooth muscle constrictors, cause mucus hypersecretion in the airways and contribute to the onset of inflammation by their ability to cause plasma extravasation and eosinophil recruitment. Indeed, cys-LTs have been recognized as among the most important mediators of asthma[8], participating both in broncho-constriction[9] and in the inflammatory component of this disease. In the latter phenomenon, the lung parenchyma plays a fundamental role[10].

Asthma is a widespread chronic disease, often of allergic/immunological origin, and its prevalence and incidence is increasing in all western countries despite the greater use of anti-asthma drugs. It is a multifactorial disease, characterized by the presence of reversible airway obstruction, inflammation and hyper-responsiveness[11]. The most significant discovery in the recent research on asthma pathophysiology has been the revelation that airway inflammation is the key component of this condition. Of the different mediators that are known to be involved in asthma, LTs are considered to be among the most potent and to play an important role in most aspects of asthma. Anti-LT compounds which inhibit either the action or the formation of these media-tors, are therefore, potential anti-asthma drugs. Indeed, LT antagonists and biosynthesis inhibitors have been developed for this purpose, and some[12] are cur-rently undergoing advanced clinical trials.

The development of novel cys-LT antagonists might be fostered by a more detailed knowledge of the receptors. Indeed, given the actual knowledge of the LT receptor model based on classical pharmacological studies both in vitro and in vivo and the fact that none of the LT receptors has been purified or cloned, the advance in develop-ing new anti-asthma drugs seems to have reached its limit.

We have addressed the problem of the characterization of *CysLT* receptors in human airways (both parenchyma and bronchi) because of the known difference between commonly used laboratory animals (guinea-pigs) and humans with regard to the receptors themselves[13,14] and to their mechanisms of signal transduction[15,16]. Particular attention has been devoted to elucidating whether in human airways, as in guinea pig[13], LTC_4 and LTD_4 have different receptors, and to the role of Ca^{2+} as a second messenger in their signal transduction pathway.

IUPHAR *cysLT* RECEPTOR CLASSIFICATION

At present, firm evidence has been obtained only for the existence of two classes of LT receptor, *CysLT$_1$* and *CysLT$_2$*, defined by a IUPHAR (International Union of Pharmacologists) panel on the basis of antagonist selectivity (Figure 1). *CysLT$_1$* receptors (Figure 1) are blocked by a series of classical antagonists of different structural types and by BAY u9773; *CysLT$_2$* are receptors not blocked by classical antagonists, but are blocked by BAY u9773[17,18]. Thus, BAY u9773 is currently the only 'dual' antagonist that clearly has activity at both *CysLT$_1$* and *CysLT$_2$* receptors[19–21]. The existence of a third class of receptors, namely *CysLT$_3$*, has been proposed recently[22]: this is resistant to both classical antagonists and BAY u9773, and has not yet been recognized by IUPHAR.

STUDIES IN HUMAN AIRWAYS

Functional studies

Functional data suggested that human bronchi do not contain different *CysLT* receptors for LTC_4 and LTD_4: bronchoconstriction elicited by LTC_4 or LTD_4 cannot be discriminated using either the antagonist FPL55712[14] or other more potent and selective cys-LT antagonists[12,23]. Thus, the receptors on human bronchi seem to recognize LTC_4 and LTD_4 equally well. and must be classified as *CysLT$_1$* as they are sensitive to both classical antagonists and BAY u9773[20]. The situation seems quite different in human lung parenchyma. LTC_4 and LTD_4 have been demonstrated to contract strips from human lung parenchyma under metabolically controlled conditions, but no clear-cut results are available to classify the receptors involved[24].

This is at variance with the results obtained in guinea-pig trachea. Cuthbert and

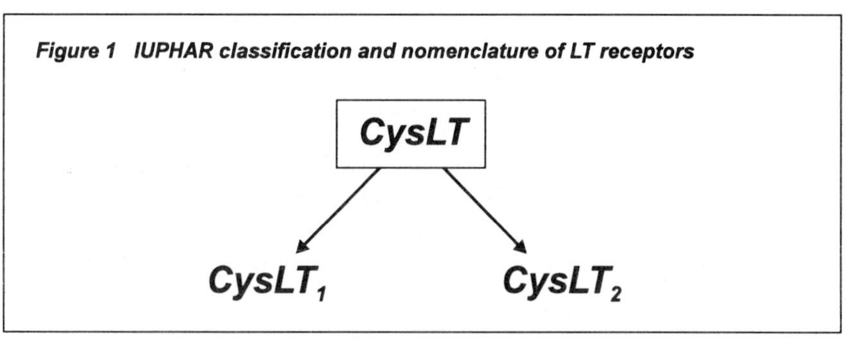

Figure 1   IUPHAR classification and nomenclature of LT receptors

coworkers[19] identified two different classes of *CysLT* receptors in this tissue and classified them as *CysLT₁* (predominantly activated by LTD₄/LTE₄) and *CysLT₂* (predominantly activated by LTC₄).

Binding studies in human lung parenchyma

Few reports on the identification of LTD_4 receptors in human airways by means of binding studies have appeared in the literature[25-27]. LTC_4 binds to a variety of non-receptor sites, e.g. enzymes involved in its synthesis and metabolism, and transporters[28-30]. So far, such binding proteins have impaired the identification of specific receptors by ligand-binding studies. For this reason, we have performed binding studies with $[^3H]LTC_4$ and $[^3H]$ LTD_4 in the absence and presence of *S*-decyl-glutathione (*S*-decyl-GSH), a high affinity ligand for non-receptor LTC_4 binding sites[31] which is devoid of either agonist or antagonist activities[32,33]. *S*-decyl-GSH was able to unmask a high affinity binding site for LTC_4 with receptor characteristics in membranes from human lung parenchyma[34,35].

Computerized analysis[36,37] of the equilibrium binding curves for $[^3H]$ LTC_4 and $[^3H]$ LTD_4 in the presence of *S*-decyl-GSH demonstrated the existence of two different classes of binding sites for each of these LTs (K_d 0.015 and 105 nM for LTC_4; 0.023 and 230 nM for LTD_4). The sites more specific for LTD_4 displayed features typical of G-protein coupled receptors. Thus, they are interconverted by stable GTP analogues and are sensitive to divalent cations. This does not apply to LTC_4 sites. These data support the hypothesis of the existence of distinct binding sites (possibly receptors) for LTC_4 and LTD_4. However, both agonists, besides interacting with its own receptor, interacted also with the other one, albeit with an affinity many hundred-fold lower than that for its own site (Figure 2).

In addition, a number of antagonists (ICI 198,615, SKF 104353, Ro 24–5913, MK-571) displayed at least 2–3 orders of magnitude differences in affinities for the proteins labelled by $[^3H]$ LTC_4 or $[^3H]$ LTD_4. In particular, these antagonists displayed K_ds in the μM range against $[^3H]$ LTC_4 and up to 100-fold lower values against $[^3H]$ LTD_4. Once again, this suggests the existence of distinct receptors for LTC_4 and LTD_4.

LTD₄ signal transduction in smooth muscle cells from human bronchi

In order to investigate the transduction mechanisms for LTD_4, we have used human bronchial cells, because of the high degree of heterogeneity of the parenchymal tissue. We have set up a cultured smooth muscle cell line obtained from macroscopically normal human bronchi and we have characterized it by means of a monoclonal antibody to α-actin, which is characteristic of smooth muscle cells.

These cells responded to histamine, acetylcholine, bradykinin and LTD_4 with morphological changes compatible with the onset of contraction, as demonstrated by light and electron microscopy. Thus, these smooth muscle cells possess receptors for the most important mediators of bronchoconstriction and represent a good model to study the signal transduction pathways involved in asthma.

Using the fluorescent probe Fluo 3[38], we demonstrated that a population of the bronchial cells responded to histamine, acetylcholine and bradykinin with a marked increase in $[Ca^{2+}]_i$ (3- to 8-fold over basal; Figure 3). The response was antagonized

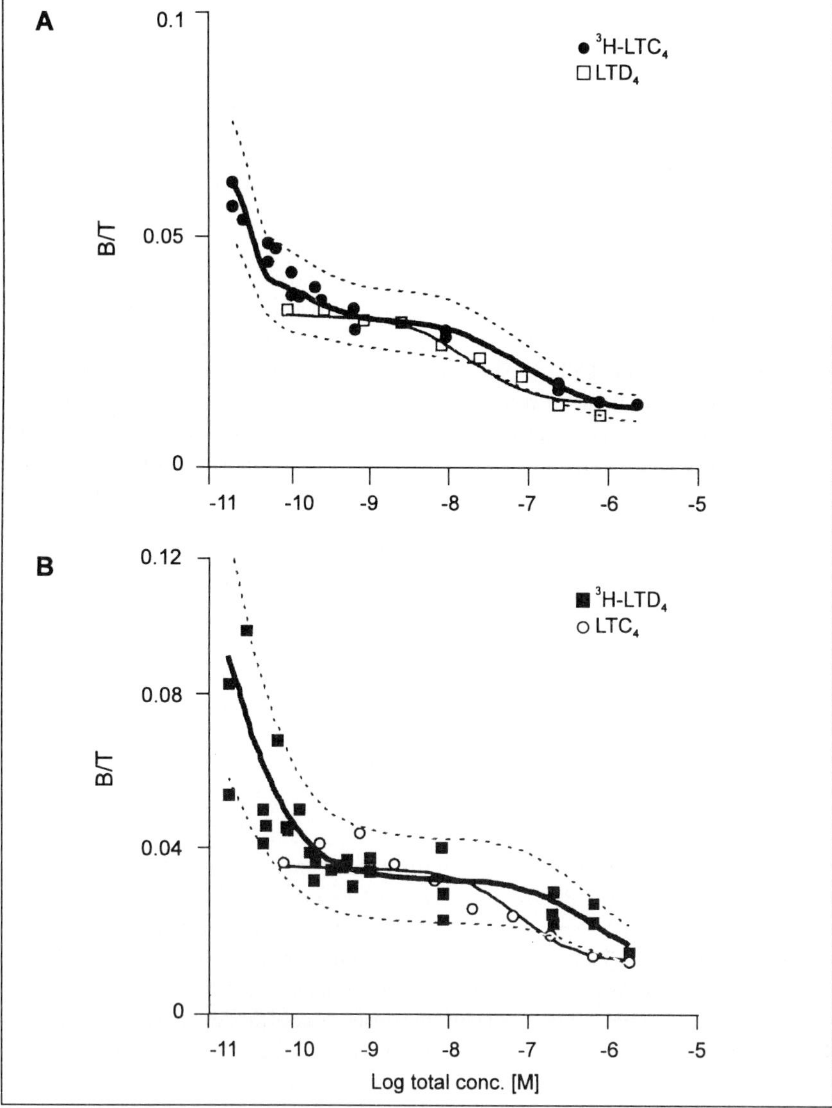

Figure 2 *Homologous and heterologous curves of [³H] LTC$_4$ and [³H] LTD$_4$ in membranes from human lung parenchyma. (A) Mixed type curve of [³H] LTC$_4$ (●) and heterologous competition curves of LTD$_4$ (□). (B) Mixed type curve of [³H] LTD$_4$ (■) and heterologous competition curves of LTC$_4$ (○). Dotted lines represent ± 95% confidence limits and are shown only for the control curve, for the sake of clarity*

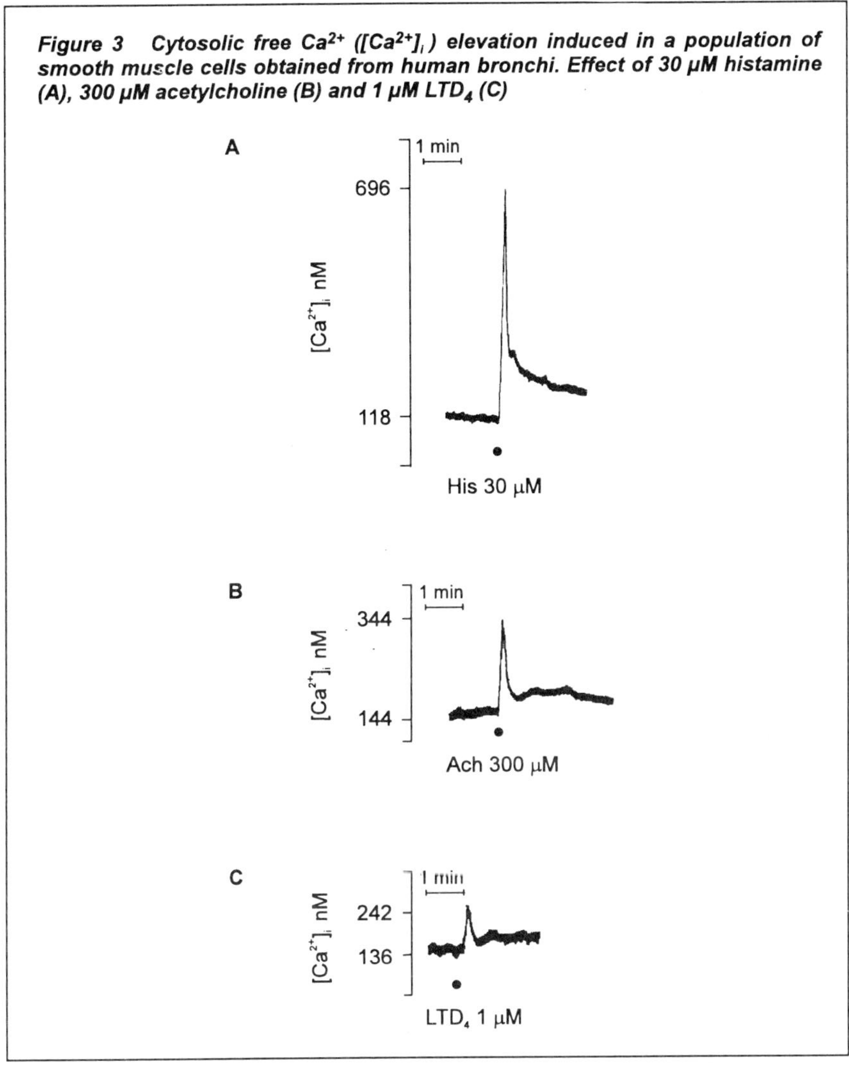

Figure 3   *Cytosolic free Ca²⁺ ([Ca²⁺]ᵢ) elevation induced in a population of smooth muscle cells obtained from human bronchi. Effect of 30 μM histamine (A), 300 μM acetylcholine (B) and 1 μM LTD₄ (C)*

by the specific antagonists mepyramine, atropine and HOE 140, respectively. On the contrary, LTD_4 was only able to elicit a very modest, if any, $[Ca^{2+}]i$ transient (Figure 3). This result was rather unexpected on the basis of the evidence obtained in other tissues[39,40]. Even when $[Ca^{2+}]$ variations were assessed at the single cell level by means of laser confocal microscopy, the LTD_4 trigger response was on average lower than that of histamine.

In the search for a Ca^{2+}-independent alternative signal transduction pathway, we investigated the activation of different isoforms of protein kinase (PK) C. Activation was assessed by means of polyclonal antibodies used to analyse SDS-PAGE separation of total, cytosolic and particulate fractions, thus quantitating the translocation of the PKC isoforms. LTD_4 was able to activate PKCε a calcium-independent isoform, and this translocation was specifically inhibited by the antagonist SKF 104353. At variance with these results, histamine was able to activate specifically the calcium-dependent isoform PKCα. Thus, the signal transduction for LTD_4 in human bronchi is at least partially Ca^{2+}-independent.

CONCLUSIONS

The available literature[19,20], as well as data obtained in our laboratory, indicate that additional classes and subclasses of *CysLT* receptors might exist, in addition to those officially recognized by IUPHAR. Indeed, the IUPHAR committee itself recognizes that the present classification is almost certainly an over-simplification[41]. Thus, as we have recently pointed out[42], we would like to suggest that, within each class of *CysLT* receptors (*CysLT$_1$*, *CysLT$_2$* and perhaps even *CysLT$_3$*) different subtypes of receptors might exist, which can be distinguished on the basis of their preference, or lack of it, for a single agonist. For example, in human lung parenchyma *CysLT$_1$* would recognize LTD_4 preferentially, while a different receptor such as *CysLT$_2$* and *CysLT$_3$* would mainly recognize LTC_4. Given the potential problems one might encounter when using agonists to define receptor subtypes (including the heterogeneity of tissues and species differences)[43], the validity of this hypothesis will have to await cloning of the receptors.

As far as the signal transduction pathway is concerned, in human lung parenchyma the LTD_4 receptor is coupled to G-proteins, while the putative LTC_4 receptor is not. Furthermore, in human bronchi Ca^{2+} is not the sole second messenger involved in the response, the Ca^{2+}-insensitive PKCε is also activated in response to LTD_4.

References

1. Drazen JM, Austen KF. Leukotrienes and airway responses. Am Rev Resp Dis. 1987; 135: 333–7.
2. Lewis RA, Robin JL. Arachidonic acid derivatives as mediators of asthma. J Allergy Clin Immunol. 1985; 76: 259–64.
3. Thien FCK, Walters EH. Eicosanoids and asthma: An update. Prostaglandins Leukot Essent Fatty Acids. 1995; 52: 271–88.
4. Feinmark SJ, Cannon PJ. Endothelial cell leukotriene C_4 synthesis results from intercellular transfer of leukotriene A_4 synthesized by polymorphonuclear leukocytes. J Biol Chem. 1986; 261: 16466–72.
5. Maclouf J, Murphy RC, Henson P. Transcellular sulfidopeptide leukotriene biosynthetic capacity of vascular cells. Blood. 1989; 74: 703–7.
6. Feinmark SJ. Leukotriene C_4 biosynthesis during polymorphonuclear leukocyte-vascular cell interactions. Methods Enzymol. 1990; 187: 559–67.
7. Maclouf J, Murphy RC. Transcellular metabolism of neutrophil-derived leukotriene A_4 by human platelets. J Biol Chem. 1988; 263: 174–81.
8. Piper PJ, Conroy DM, Costello JF, et al. Leukotrienes and inflammatory lung disease. Ann NY Acad Sci USA. 1991; 629: 112–19.
9. Dahlén SE, Hedqvist P, Hammarström S, Samuelsson B. Leukotrienes are potent constrictors of human bronchi. Nature. 1980; 288: 484–6.

10. Chanarin N, Johnston SL. Leukotrienes as a target in asthma therapy. Drugs. 1994; 47: 12–24.

11. Barnes PJ. New aspects of asthma. J Int Med. 1992; 231: 453–61.

12. Salmon JA, Garland LG. Leukotriene antagonists and inhibitors of leukotriene biosynthesis as potential therapeutic agents. Prog Drug Res. 1991; 37: 9–90.

13. Snyder DW, Krell RD. Pharmacological evidence for a distinct leukotriene C_4 receptor in guinea-pig trachea. J Pharmacol Exp Ther. 1984; 231: 616–22.

14. Buckner CK, Krell RD, Laravuso RB, Coursin DB, Bernstein PR, Will JA. Pharmacogical evidence that human intralobar airways do not contain different receptors that mediate contractions to leukotriene C_4 and leukotriene D_4. J Pharmacol Exp Ther. 1986; 237: 558–62.

15. Sautebin L, Viganò T, Grassi E, et al. Release of leukotrienes, induced by the Ca++ ionophore A23187, from human lung parenchyma in vitro. J Pharmacol Exp Ther. 1985; 234: 217–21.

16. Folco GC, Hansson G, Granström E. Leukotriene C_4 stimulates TXA_2 formation in isolated sensitized guinea-pig lungs. Biochem Pharmacol. 1981; 30: 2591–3.

17. Coleman RA, Eglen RM, Jones RL, et al. Prostanoid and leukotriene receptors: a progress report from the IUPHAR working parties on classification and nomenclature. Adv Prostaglandin, Thromboxane, Leukotriene Res. 1995; 23: 283–5.

18. Watson S, Girdlestone D. TiPS receptor and ion channel nomenclature. Supplement 1996. Trends Pharmacol Sci. 1996; 45–6.

19. Cuthbert NJ, Tudhope SR, Gardiner PJ, et al. BAY u9773 an LTC_4 antagonist in the guinea pig trachea. Ann NY Acad Sci. 1991; 629: 402–4.

20. Labat C, Ortiz JL, Norel X, et al. A second cysteinyl leukotriene receptor in human lung. J Pharmacol Exp Ther. 1992; 263: 800–5.

21. Gardiner PJ, Abram TS, Tudhope SR, Cuthbert NJ, Norman P, Brink C. Leukotriene receptors and their selective antagonists. Adv Prostaglandin, Thromboxane, Leukotriene Res. 1994; 22: 49–61.

22. Tudhope SR, Cuthbert NJ, Abram TS, et al. BAY u9773, a novel antagonist of cysteinyl leukotrienes with activity against two receptor subtypes. Eur J Pharmacol. 1994; 264: 317–23.

23. Brooks CDW, Summers JB. Modulators of leukotriene biosynthesis and receptor activation. J Med Chem. 1996; 39: 2629–54.

24. Gardiner PJ, Cuthbert NJ. Characterisation of the leukotriene receptor(s) on human isolated lung strips. Agents Actions Suppl. 1988; 23: 121–8.

25. Lewis MA, Mong S, Vessella RL, Crooke ST. Identification and characterization of leukotriene D_4 receptors in adult and fetal human lung. Biochem Pharmacol. 1985; 34: 4311–7.

26. Aharony D, Falcone RC. Binding of ^{3}H-LTD$_4$ and the peptide leukotriene antagonist ^{3}H-ICI 198,615 to receptors on human lung membranes. In: Zor U, Naor Z, Danon A, editors. Leukotrienes and Prostanoids in Health and Disease. Basel: Karger, 1989: 67–71.

27. Rovati GE, Giovanazzi S, Mezzetti M, Nicosia S. Heterogeneity of binding sites for ^{3}H-ICI 198,615 in human lung parenchyma. Biochem Pharmacol. 1992; 44: 1411–15.

28. Metters KM, Sawyer N, Nicholson DW. Microsomal glutathione S-transferase is the predominantly leukotriene C_4 binding site in cellular membranes. J Biol Chem. 1994; 269: 12816–23.

29. Nicholson DW, Ali A, Klemba MW, Munday NA, Zamboni RJ, Ford-Hutchinson AW. Human leukotriene C_4 synthase expression in dimethyl sulfoxide-differentiated U937 cells. J Biol Chem. 1992; 267: 17849–57.

30. Keppler D. Leukotrienes: Biosynthesis, transport, inactivation, and analysis. Rev Physiol Biochem Pharmacol. 1992; 121: 1–30.

31. Ishikawa T, Kobayashi K, Sogame Y, Hayashi K. Evidence for leukotriene C_4 transport mediated by an ATP-dependent glutathione S-conjugate carrier in rat heart and liver plasma membranes. FEBS Lett. 1989; 259: 95–8.

32. Norman P, Abram TS, Kluender HC, Gardiner PJ, Cuthbert NJ. The binding of [^{3}H]leukotriene C_4 to guinea-pig lung membranes. The lack of correlation of LTC_4 functional activity with binding affinity. Eur J Pharmacol. 1987; 143: 323–34.

33. Sala A, Civelli M, Oliva D, et al. Contractile and binding activities of structural analogues of LTC_4 in the longitudinal muscle of guinea-pig ileum. Eicosanoids. 1990; 3: 105–10.
34. Nicosia S, Capra V, Accomazzo MR, et al. Receptors and second messengers for Cys-leukotrienes. In: Folco GC, Samuelsson B, Maclouf J, Velo GP, editors. Eicosanoids From Biotechnology to Therapeutic Application. New York and London: Plenum Press, 1996: 127–36.
35. Capra V, Nicosia S, Ragnini D, Mezzetti M, Keppler D, Rovati GE. Identification and characterization of two Cys-leukotriene high-affinity binding sites with receptor characteristics in human lung parenchyma. Mol Pharmacol. 1998 (in press).
36. Rovati GE, Rabin D, Munson PJ. Analysis, design and optimization of ligand binding experiments. In: Maggi M, Geenen EV, editors. Horizons in Endocrinology (Vol II). New York: Serono Symposia Publication from Raven Press, vol 76, 1991: 155–67.
37. Rovati GE. Rational design and analysis for ligand binding studies: Tricks, tips and pitfalls. Pharmacol Res. 1993; 28: 277–99.
38. Kao JP, Harootunian AT, Tsien RY. Photochemically generated cytosolic calcium pulses and their detection by fluo-3. J Biol Chem. 1989; 264: 8179–84.
39. Oliva D, Accomazzo MR, Giovanazzi S, Nicosia S. Correlation between leukotriene D_4-induced contraction and cytosolic calcium elevation: a quantitative and simultaneous evaluation in smooth muscle. J Pharm Exp Ther. 1994; 268: 159–66.
40. Crooke ST, Mattern M. Sarau HM, et al. The signal transduction system of the leukotriene D_4 receptor. Trends Pharmacol Sci. 1989; 10: 103–7.
41. Coleman RA. Compendium from the IUPHAR Committee for leukotriene receptor classification. 1994 distributed by the 9th International Conference on Prostaglandin and Related Compounds, Florence (Italy).
42. Rovati GE, Capra V, Nicosia S. More on the classification of cysteinyl leukotriene receptors. Trends Pharmacol Sci. 1997; 18: 148.
43. Kenakin TP, Bond RA, Bonner TI. Definition of pharmacological receptors. Pharm Rev. 1992; 44: 351–62.

5 How to measure leukotrienes in man

M. KUMLIN

The involvement of leukotrienes (LTs) in asthma mainly concerns the cysteinyl-leukotrienes (cys-LTs, LTC_4, D_4 and E_4), which are chemical mediators of events in the airways as part of an asthmatic attack[1]. There is still a debate in the literature whether the proinflammatory compound LTB_4, formed from the common unstable epoxide intermediate LTA_4, also contributes to the airway inflammation associated with asthma[2].

This chapter will focus primarily on measurements of the cys-LTs. Sensitive, specific, reproducible and simple analytical tools for measurements of leukotrienes in man are needed for several applications. The evaluation of anti-leukotrienes as new anti-asthmatic drugs requires investigations in which these compounds can be accurately measured. It is of interest to measure in vitro as well as in vivo production of LTs in order to achieve extended knowledge of their involvement in a number of pathological disorders. Analyses of LTs in tissues and cells reflect in vitro biosynthesis, whereas measurements of metabolites in different biological fluids may be used as index of in vivo release of the compounds[3].

MEASUREMENTS IN LUNG TISSUE AND CELLS FROM THE AIRWAYS

Biosynthesis of eicosanoids can be studied in vitro by incubation of cells and tissues in the presence of stimuli of the release and enzymatic conversion of arachidonic acid. By this means cell specific and transcellular formation of mediators can be studied. Intermediates such as the epoxide LTA_4 can be added as a substrate to explore further cell or tissue specific metabolism into LTC_4 and/or LTB_4. However, the results from in vitro studies do not always reflect in vivo release in response to challenge. Furthermore, the use of invasive techniques is necessary to obtain the material and access to suitable tissue samples from patients with asthma is limited.

A number of studies have documented ionophore or anti-IgE-induced release of mediators from lung tissue, biopsy specimens or cells from the airways. The cys-LTs were shown to be formed in human lung cells in vitro[4], and in a comprehensive study on LT formation in chopped human lung, an anti-IgE mediated release of specifically the cys-LTs was demonstrated[5]. Allergen-induced formation of cys-LTs was likewise demonstrated in rare samples of lung tissue from patients with atopic asthma[6].

MEASUREMENT IN NASAL AND BRONCHOALVEOLAR LAVAGE FLUIDS

Cell counts and mediator release into the airways under basal conditions and in response to challenge may be assessed in nasal (NAL)[7,8] or bronchoalveolar lavage fluids (BAL)[9-11]. By this means a direct picture of events in the airways can be obtained and the cell profile may serve to complement the pattern of released mediators. Lavage fluids are not easy to obtain, however, with the consequence that generally only a limited number of subjects or samples has been studied. Furthermore, since the recovery of lavage fluid may differ, the true concentration of mediators is not always possible to predict[12]. It is also debatable as to what metabolites are the most suitable targets for analysis in lavage fluids. The breakdown of the mediators must be considered and, depending on the time passing between challenge and lavage, different metabolites will be present in the fluids[12,13].

Release of mediators into the alveolar space may also be analysed after a local challenge via the bronchoscope[13,14]. Endobronchial challenge with allergen[13] or aspirin[14] led to increased levels of leukotrienes and other eicosanoids in BAL fluid. Mediator release in the mucosa of the airways has also been estimated by analysis in nasopharyngeal or tracheobronchial secretions[15,16].

MEASUREMENT OF CIRCULATING METABOLITES IN BLOOD, SERUM OR PLASMA

Monitoring circulating metabolites of LTs in whole blood or plasma could be one approach to measure in vivo production. Blood samples can easily be taken without disturbance of the airway function in patients with asthma or other obstructive lung diseases. Invasive techniques are, however, involved in the collection of samples which bring about a high risk of artifactual ex vivo formation of compounds due to activation of cells during sampling[17]. Cumbersome purification procedures may also be required. More important is the fact that concentrations of circulating LTs is below the detection limit of most assays used to date[18,19]. Detectable levels of immunoreactive LTC_4 have been reported in plasma of asthmatic patients[20,21], but considering the rapid clearance of LTs from the bloodstream, the renal clearance and the concentrations of LTE_4 in urine, it appears unlikely that a level above 100 pg/ml is actually a true reflection of circulating concentration of cys-LTs.

MEASUREMENT IN URINE

Urine is a biological fluid that is easy to collect with no significant risk of artifactual formation of LTs. The non-invasive sampling procedure also makes repeated collection possible from patients with different types of respiratory diseases, and the pattern of metabolites in urine probably reflects the whole body production. Furthermore, in contrast to the difficulties in determining concentrations of mediators in NAL and BAL fluids discussed above, the concentrations of urinary metabolites may be related to the constant excretion of creatinine to correct for diuresis variations, and thus obtain true reflections of changes in the in vivo mediator release[22].

It is, however, important to remember that liver and kidney disorders affect the urinary excretion of LT metabolites and that such data may be misinterpreted as altered in vivo production[23,24]. For instance, a marked increase of renal cys-LT excretion was observed in patients with liver cirrhosis[25]. Since the liver is the major organ which metabolizes and eliminates cys-LTs into bile, the increased urinary excretion of LTE_4 in cirrhosis patients is probably due to a reduced functional liver mass[25]. A defect in the ATP-dependent transport mechanism for cys-LTs in liver membranes[26], and bile duct obstruction[27] may likewise result in increased urinary excretion of LTE_4 with or without an altered in vivo production of LTC_4.

In order to decide which metabolite to measure in urine we need to know the metabolic fate of the LTs in vivo. The pulmonary metabolism of LTC_4 in vitro results in a rapid, almost exclusive formation of LTE_4 with no further conversion, and thus LTE_4 seems to be the end product of cys-LTs in the lung[5].

A few studies have focused on the in vivo metabolism of cys-LTs following administration of LTC_4 or LTD_4 intravenously[28–31], by inhalation[32] or after endogenous formation in response to allergen challenge[33]. A similar proportion, generally about 5%, of exogenously supplied LTs was recovered as intact LTE_4 in the urine. Together all these studies suggest that LTE_4, being a major urinary metabolite, is suitable as a target for measurements of in vivo production of cys-LTs[29–32,34]. Metabolism of bronchoconstrictor doses of inhaled LTC_4 or LTE_4 in patients with asthma strongly supports the use of urinary LTE_4 as an index specifically reflecting cys-LT release in the airways of asthmatics[35].

An important question is, of course, the stability of LTE_4 in the urine from the time of sampling to the time of analysis. Antioxidants are often added to the urine to prevent oxidation or breakdown of LTs. We investigated whether the presence of the antioxidant 4-hydroxy-TEMPO free radical (1 mM) and a pH of 9 influences the stability of LTE_4 in buffer and urine stored at -20°C[22]. If anything, the relative amount of intact LTE_4 after 2 months tended to be less in the samples with preservatives. In buffer this phenomenon was even more pronounced[22]. In agreement with this, we recovered more than 90% of LTE_4 immunoreactivity after about 10 months' storage of urine samples at -20°C without any additions. Interestingly, it was recently demonstrated that LTE_4 is stable even at room temperature for at least 24 h[36].

A peak increase in urinary LTE_4, as a result of provoked release of LTs is generally fairly short lasting[22,34,37]. In order to trap such a transient increase, collection of urine with short intervals is necessary. We applied EIA analysis to urine samples collected hourly during bronchial provocation with a single dose of allergen. There was a significant post-challenge peak increase in urinary LTE_4 within 1 h of the allergen-induced airway obstruction, with values returning to pre-challenge levels within the next few hours. When mean values of samples collected at 2–4 h intervals were defined as the post-challenge level, the calculated mean increase from baseline did not reach statistical significance after 2 h[38]. The importance of frequent sampling is further illustrated by the peak increase in urinary LTE_4 detected 1.5 h after inhalation of LTC_4 or LTE_4 in asthmatics, the levels of LTE_4 returning almost back to baseline by 3.5 h[35].

When bronchial provocations were performed cumulatively, with increasing doses of allergen given to the patient[39], a likewise significant post-challenge increase in urinary LTE_4 was seen within 2 h of the allergen-induced airway obstruction. When patients were pretreated with the LT receptor antagonist zafirlukast, the tolerance for allergen was increased, with an approximate 5-fold increase in PD_{20}, and the post-challenge mean increase in urinary LTE_4 excretion was enhanced. This indicates a dose-dependent release of LTs in response to the allergen challenge[34].

To explore further the mechanism behind the allergen-induced LT release we compared the results from the single dose challenge with cumulative challenge with allergen. The mean pre-challenge levels of urinary LTE_4 were the same on both occasions, whereas post-challenge levels after cumulative challenge were significantly higher than those seen when the same total dose of allergen was given as a single administration[38]. Thus, in addition to a dose-dependent release, repeated challenge, and perhaps a longer time for activation of the inflammatory cells producing the LTs, seems to be factors which determine the amount of LTs excreted into the urine. The protocol used for bronchial provocation may, therefore, significantly influence the results from analysis of urinary LTE_4 in studies of induced asthma.

METHODS FOR MEASUREMENTS OF URINARY LTE_4

Immunoassays based on radioactivity (RIA) or enzyme activity (EIA) are regarded as rapid and sensitive methods suitable for analysis of different eicosanoids[40]. A number of antibodies to cys-LTs with different specificity are commercially available. Analyses by EIA or RIA have been most commonly performed in combination with reverse phase-high performance liquid chromatography (RP-HPLC)[11,41,42]. To follow endogenous production of cys-LTs we have validated an EIA for LTE_4[22]. The assay is routinely used in unpurified urine samples with random comparisons with results from the same samples after purification on solid phase extraction (SPE) and RP-HPLC and have proved to be reliable. Recently, an alternative purification method using immunofiltration prior to immunoassay was described as a less time-consuming alternative to purification on HPLC[36]. Measurements of urinary LTE_4 with RP-HPLC alone is not an alternative due to the low sensitivity of the detection with ultra-violet absorbance.

Gas chromatography-mass spectrometry (GC-MS) is a highly sensitive and specific method and could theoretically be an alternative for the measurement of urinary LTE_4. However, it has not been possible to apply derivatization procedures used for other eicosanoids prior to GC-MS to cys-LTs. Recently, an alternative GC-MS method was described in which the cys-LTs were subjected to catalytic reduction and desulphurization prior to conversion into the pentafluorobenzyl (PFB) ester, trimethylsilyl (TMS) ether derivatives[43]. Analysis with GC-MS was subsequently performed with selected ion monitoring (SIM) using stable isotope-labelled LTE_4 analogues as internal standards. Interestingly, the values obtained with quantitative GC-MS for basal urinary LTE_4 in healthy subjects[43] correlated well with values reported from immunoassay analyses[41,44–51]. This indeed supports the reliability and usefulness of immunoassays. All mass spectrometric procedures demand cumbersome and time-consuming purification of the samples. Although GC-MS is an important tool to reliably quantify urinary LTE_4 and may serve as a gold standard for calibration of other analytical methods, it is unlikely that GC-MS will become useful for high throughput routine purposes.

URINARY LTE$_4$ IN PATIENTS WITH ASTHMA

As indicated above, urine has been found useful for measuring whole body production of the cys-LTs[11,23,34,41,42,47,52,53] and in vivo formation of cys-LTs has been documented in association with allergen-induced airway obstruction[34,41,53].

So far, a few studies have focused on basal renal excretion of LTE_4 in healthy individuals in comparison with asthmatics, and thus knowledge in this area is quite limited. Urinary excretion of LTE_4 was followed in samples collected every third hour for a period of 24 h from a group of healthy, non-asthmatic individuals and there were no signs of a diurnal variation[22]. This result has been confirmed by Asano and co-workers in healthy subjects and extended to include patients with asthma[54]. Whether there is diurnal variation in patients with nocturnal asthma is still not clear. It has been reported that patients experiencing nocturnal exacerbations showed increased excretion of urinary LTE_4 during the night, with a linear correlation between a morning dip in lung function and the urinary levels of LTE_4[55]. However, in another study the difference in urinary LTE_4 between day and night in patients with nocturnal asthma was not significant[56].

Baseline values given in the literature for patients with asthma and healthy individuals vary somewhat, mainly because different assay procedures have been used. Nevertheless, the studies generally show no significant discrepancies between baseline urinary LTE_4 in healthy non-asthmatics and in atopic asthmatics[22,47,55]. Recent studies point to higher baseline values in limited groups of patients with mild to moderate asthma[54] or subjects with nocturnal asthma[56] than in non-asthmatic individuals.

We and others have shown that aspirin-intolerant asthmatics (AIA)[57] have higher basal levels of LTE_4 in their morning urine than do aspirin-tolerant asthmatics (ATA)[22,34,50,58]. Aspirin desensitization of patients with AIA resulted in a reduced aspirin-induced increase in urinary LTE_4, whereas the basal levels in some cases even increased[59]. These findings suggest a specific importance of cys-LTs in aspirin-induced asthma.

A number of studies has now been published on release of LTs in induced asthma, and a few studies have been reported on patients presenting in the emergency room with spontaneous asthmatic attacks. On admission to the hospital, a group of subjects with acute asthma had higher urinary LTE_4 levels than control groups[11,52]. As lung function recovered, the urinary LTE_4 concentration declined to levels observed in non-asthmatics[52]. Significantly higher levels were also documented in a group of subjects experiencing spontaneous acute airway obstruction, with the highest levels found in a subgroup who readily responded to inhaled β-agonists[42]. Leukotrienes may also be involved in anaphylactic reactions without asthmatic symptoms, as judged by a significant increase in urinary excretion of LTs[60].

An increased excretion of urinary LTE_4 after allergen-induced airway obstruction was initially documented by Taylor et al.[52], and has been confirmed by us and others[33,34,53,61–63]. Studies reported in the literature have been performed according to different protocols, but nevertheless the increase in urinary LTE_4 after allergen challenge has mostly been between 2- and 5-fold in a number of independent reports[34,46,52,53]. Increased excretion of urinary LTE_4 has also been documented in association with aspirin-induced airway obstruction provoked by oral as well as inhaled routes of aspirin administration[34,50,58,59,64–67]. This reaction is exclusive to intolerant patients, since aspirin-tolerant asthmatics do not react with either bronchial obstruction or increased excretion of urinary LTE_4 in response to aspirin provocation[34].

Another interesting trigger factor in asthma is exercise. Studies of exercise-induced bronchoconstriction have produced somewhat contradictory results regarding the role of LTs. It has not yet been possible to document increased excretion of LTE_4 after exercise-induced airway obstruction[46,68], with the exception of one report on elevated urinary LTE_4 levels following exercise challenge in a group of children[69]. The role of cys-LTs in this type of asthma can therefore at present not be determined solely on the basis of analyses of urinary LTE_4. However, since several different anti-leukotriene drugs provide significant protection in exercise-induced asthma, it has been suggested that LTs also mediate this type of airway obstruction[70–73]. In fact, since exercise-induced airway obstruction is relatively short-lasting, the brief stimulation by exercise may be insufficient to generate enough LTs to be detectable above basal levels. This further suggests that the duration of a challenge contributes to the amounts of LTE_4 excreted in the urine.

Whether urinary LTE_4 is also increased in association with late phase asthmatic responses (LAR) is also somewhat unclear. A limited number of bronchial provocation studies has considered the role of LTs in LAR. Generally, a prolonged elevation of the urinary levels of LTE_4 has been documented, rather than a significant distinct second peak of increase[33,45,46,48,49,52,53,63]. Whether this is a reflection of a second phase of LT release or only reflects a continuous excretion of LTs previously formed during the early asthmatic response (EAR) has been difficult to resolve and contradictory results have been presented[48,49,53,61]. However, the rapid metabolic clearance of cys-LTs[29,31] rather supports de novo formation of LTs also during the late phase. Recent data from our laboratory support the release of cys-LTs during allergen-induced LAR in dual responders[74,75]. Involvement of LTs in LAR is further supported by pharmacological evidence: a significant attenuation of the reaction was seen after pretreatment with the LT receptor antagonist zafirlukast, alone or in combination with the histamine antagonist loratidine[76]. These latter data confirm earlier reports of significant attenuation of the LAR by antileukotriene drugs[45,61,77].

MEASUREMENT OF LTB$_4$

Since measurement of LTB_4 is not the primary focus in this chapter this will just be briefly mentioned. Knowledge of the whole body metabolism of LTB_4 is still limited and there are no methods available for routine analysis of LTB_4 metabolites in the urine. Metabolites formed in leukocytes[78] or in macrophages and lung tissue[79,80] have not been shown to be excreted in the urine. Therefore, a common approach to measure in vivo formation of LTB_4 has been to assess ex vivo ionophore-stimulated formation in leukocytes. This has been specifically used in studies with LT biosynthesis inhibitors[62,81]. In general, data obtained from such studies point to inhibition of ionophore-induced ex vivo formation of LTB_4 in leukocytes by LT biosynthesis inhibitors seems to correlate with plasma concentration of drugs rather than inhibition of airway responses[62].

MEASUREMENT OF THE PROSTAGLANDIN D_2 METABOLITE $9\alpha,11\beta$-PROSTAGLANDIN F_2

It is established that allergen challenge acts on, and provokes mediator release from, the mast cells. This makes the mast cell the most likely candidate as the cell source for cys-LT release in association with at least the early phase of allergen-induced airway obstruction. However, the mechanism behind aspirin-induced LT release in patients with aspirin-intolerant asthma is less clear. The concept of monitoring the PGD_2 metabolite $9\alpha,11\beta$-PGF_2 as a marker of mast cell activation has been introduced[82]. PGD_2 is almost exclusively formed in mast cells and $9\alpha,11\beta$-PGF_2 is an early appearing major urinary metabolite[83], for which we have validated an EIA for analysis in unpurified samples[82].

In a group of subjects with aspirin-intolerant asthma, bronchoconstriction was elicited by cumulative inhalation of increasing doses of lysine-aspirin, and urine was collected hourly. There was good agreement between the time-courses, and dose-dependence for urinary excretion of LTE_4 and $9\alpha,11\beta$-PGF_2, supporting the hypothesis that the mediators are derived from the same cell source, which would most likely be the mast cell in view of the release of $9\alpha,11\beta$-PGF_2[82]. However, there was no difference between basal levels of urinary $9\alpha,11\beta$-PGF_2 in aspirin-intolerant asthmatics when compared with other asthmatics, in contrast to the documented elevated basal levels of urinary LTE_4 in patients with aspirin-intolerant asthma[82]. One explanation for this discrepancy may be that the basal excretion of the two metabolites are derived from different cell sources whereas the aspirin-provoked release is mast cell derived for both compounds.

With the purpose of further exploring the mechanism behind the LAR, urinary $9\alpha,11\beta$-PGF_2 was measured in a study where the patients developed both EAR and LAR in response to allergen inhalation. The urinary excretion of the mast cell marker $9\alpha,11\beta$-PGF_2 increased significantly during both EAR and LAR. The levels did not return to baseline until after 24 h[74,75]. The data thus strongly support mast cell involvement in the LAR as well as the EAR in response to allergen.

CONCLUSIONS

For several reasons, urine seems to be the biological fluid of choice for monitoring in vivo biosynthesis of cys-LTs in man, and urinary LTE_4 can serve as a marker of pulmonary production specifically. EIA is a sensitive and specific technique for the measurement of LTE_4 with high sample capacity, and samples stored in the freezer without preservatives can be analysed with EIA without prior purification. Purification of the samples with SPE and HPLC causes substantial losses of LTs and does not necessarily improve the assay. Other methods for purification may be alternatives if they prove to be beneficial in terms of accuracy, time and cost[36]. Mild or short-lived stimulation may cause a transient increase in urinary LTE_4 that can only be detected if samples are collected on an hourly basis. Finally, the lack of diurnal variation in the excretion of urinary LTE_4 in healthy non-asthmatic subjects, and most likely in asthmatic patients without nocturnal exacerbations, increases the usefulness of analysis of urinary LTE_4 as an index of in vivo production.

The sensitive and rather simple method we describe for analysis of LTE_4 in human urine may be useful in further clinical trials with anti-leukotriene drugs as well as for diagnosis and control of treatment of asthma and airway inflammation. Furthermore, since a multitude of pathological disorders, such as other pulmonary diseases[11,84,85], atopic diseases[86], anaphylactic reactions[60], cardiovascular disorders[87,88] and autoimmune diseases[89–91], have been associated with altered excretion of urinary LTE_4, this method may become applicable in a broad range of experimental clinical studies.

References

1. Dahlén S-E. Leukotrienes and related lipoxygenase products. In: Barnes PJ, Rodger IW, Thomson NC, Barnes PJ, Thomson NC, editors. Asthma: Basic mechanisms and clinical management. London: Academic Press, 1988: 213–30.
2. Christie P, Barnes N. Leukotriene B_4 and asthma. Thorax. 1996; 12: 1171–3.
3. Kumlin M. Analytical methods for the measurements of leukotrienes and other eicosanoids in biological samples from asthmatic subjects. J Chromatography A. 1996; 725: 29–40.
4. MacGlashan DW Jr, Schleimer RP, Peters SP, et al. Generation of leukotrienes by purified human lung mast cells. J Clin Invest. 1982; 70: 747–51.
5. Kumlin M, Dahlén S-E. Characteristics of formation and further metabolism of leukotrienes in the chopped human lung. Biochim Biophys Acta. 1990; 1044: 201–10.
6. Dahlén S-E, Hansson G, Hedqvist P, Björck T, Granström E, Dahlén B. Allergen challenge of lung tissue from asthmatics elicits bronchial contraction that correlates with the release of leukotrienes C_4, D_4 and E_4. Proc Natl Acad Sci USA. 1983; 80: 1712–16.
7. Picado C, Ramis I, Rosellò J, et al. Release of peptide leukotriene into nasal secretions after local instillation of aspirin in aspirin-sensitive asthmatic patients. Am Rev Resp Dis. 1992; 145: 65–9.
8. Ramis I, Catafau JR, Serra J, Bulbena O, Picado C, Gelpi E. In vivo release of 15-HETE and other arachidonic acid metabolites in nasal secretions during early allergic reactions. Prostaglandins. 1991; 42: 411–20.
9. Lam S, Chan H, LeRiche JC, Chan-Yeung M, Salari H. Release of leukotrienes in patients with bronchial asthma. J Allergy Clin Immunol. 1988; 81: 711–17.
10. Wardlaw AJ, Hay H, Cromwell O, Collins JV, Kay AB. Leukotrienes, LTC_4 and LTB_4, in bronchoalveolar lavage in bronchial asthma and other respiratory diseases. J Allergy Clin Immunol. 1989; 84: 19–26.
11. Westcott JY, Johnston K, Batt RA, Wenzel SE, Voelkel NF. Measurement of peptidoleukotrienes in biological fluids. J Appl Physiol. 1990; 68: 2640–8.
12. Bisgaard H, Robinson C, Romeling F, Mygind N, Church M, Holgate S. Leukotriene C_4 and histamine in early allergic reaction in the nose. Allergy. 1988; 43: 219–27.
13. Wenzel SE, Larsen GL, Johnston K, Voelkel NF, Westcott JY. Elevated levels of leukotriene C_4 in bronchoalveolar lavage fluid from atopic asthmatics after endobronchial allergen challenge. Am Rev Resp Dis. 1990; 142: 112–19.
14. Szczeklik A, Sladek K, Dworski R, et al. Bronchial aspirin challenge causes specific

eicosanoid response in aspirin-sensitive asthmatics. Am J Resp Crit Care Med. 1996; 154: 1608–14.

15. Volovitz B, Osur SL, Bernstein JM, Ogra PL. Leukotriene C_4 release in upper respiratory mucosa during natural exposure to ragweed in ragweed-sensitive children. J Allergy Clin Immunol. 1988; 82: 414–18.

16. Volovitz B, Nathanson I, DeCastro G, et al. Relationship between leukotriene C_4 and an uteroglobin-like protein in nasal and tracheobronchial mucosa of children. Implication in acute respiratory illnesses. Int Arch Allergy Appl Immunol. 1988; 86: 420–5.

17. Granström E, Kumlin M. Metabolism of prostaglandins and lipoxygenase products: Relevance for eicosanoid assay. In: Benedetto C, McDonald RG, Nigam S, et al., editors. Prostaglandins and related substances: A practical approach. Oxford: IRL Press, 1987; 5–27.

18. Heavey DJ, Soberman RJ, Lewis RA, Spur B, Austen KF. Critical consideration in the development of an assay for sulfidopeptide leukotrienes in plasma. Prostaglandins. 1987; 33: 693–708.

19. Sampson AP, Castling DP, Green CP, Price JF. Persistent increase in plasma and urinary leukotrienes after acute asthma. Arch Dis Child. 1995; 73: 221–5.

20. Shiratsuki N, Uyama O, Kitada O, et al. Effects of hydrocortisone and aminophylline on plasma leukotriene C_4 levels in patients during an asthmatic attack. Prostaglandins Leukotrienes Essential Fatty Acids. 1990; 40: 285–9.

21. Schwartzberg S, Shelov S, Van Praag D. Blood leukotriene levels during the acute asthma attack in children. Prostaglandins Leukotrienes Med. 1987; 26: 143–55.

22. Kumlin M, Stensvad F, Larsson L, Dahlén B, Dahlén S-E. Validation and application of a new simple strategy for measurements of leukotriene E_4 in human urine. Clin Exp Allergy. 1995; 25: 467–79.

23. Huber M, Kästner S, Schölmerich J, Gerok W, Keppler D. Analysis of cysteinyl leukotrienes in human urine: Enhanced excretion in patients with liver cirrhosis and hepatorenal syndrome. Eur J Clin Invest. 1989; 19: 53–60.

24. Mayatepek E, Pecher G. Increased excretion of endogenous urinary leukotriene E_4 in extrahepatic cholestasis. Clin Chim Acta. 1993; 218: 185–92.

25. Uemura M, Buchholz U, Kojima H, et al. Cysteinyl leukotrienes in the urine of patients with liver diseases. Hepatology. 1994; 20: 804–12.

26. Richter L, Hesselbarth N, Eitner K, Bosseckert H, Krell H. Increased biliary secretion of cysteinyl-leukotrienes in human bile duct obstruction. J Hepatol. 1996; 25: 725–32.

27. Ishikawa T, Muller M, Klunemann C, Schaub T, Keppler D. ATP-dependent primary active transport of cysteinyl leukotrienes across liver canalicular membrane. Role of the ATP-dependent transport system for glutathione S-conjugates. J Biol Chem. 1990; 265: 19279–86.

28. Örning L, Kaijser L, Hammarström S. In vivo metabolism of leukotriene C_4 in man: Urinary excretion of leukotriene E_4. Biochem Biophys Res Commun. 1985; 130: 214–20.

29. Huber M, Müller J, Leier I, et al. Metabolism of cysteinyl leukotrienes in monkey and man. Eur J Biochem. 1990; 194: 309–15.

30. Maltby NH, Taylor GW, Ritter JM, Moore K, Fuller RW, Dollery CT. Leukotriene C_4 elimination and metabolism in man. J Allergy Clin Immunol. 1990; 85: 3–9.

31. Sala A, Voelkel N, Maclouf J, Murphy RC. Leukotriene E_4 elimination and metabolism in normal human subjects. J Biol Chem. 1990; 265: 21771–8.

32. Verhagen J, Bel EH, Kijne GM, Sterk PJ, Bruynzeel PLB, Veldink GA, Vliegenthart JFG. The excretion of leukotriene E_4 into urine following inhalation of leukotriene D_4 by human individuals. Biochem Biophys Res Commun. 1987; 148: 864–8.

33. Tagari P, Rasmussen JB, Delorme D, et al. Comparison of urinary leukotriene E_4 and 16-carboxytetranordihydro leukotriene E_4 excretion in allergic asthmatics after inhaled antigen. Eicosanoids. 1990; 3: 75–80.

34. Kumlin M, Dahlén B, Björck T, Zetterström O, Granström E, Dahlén S-E. Urinary excretion of leukotriene E_4 and 11-dehydro-thromboxane B_2 in response to bronchial provocations with allergen, aspirin, leukotriene D_4, and histamine in asthmatics. Am Rev Resp Dis. 1992; 146: 96–103.

35. Christie PE, Tagari P, Ford-Hutchinson AW, et al. Increased urinary LTE_4 excretion following inhalation of LTC_4 and LTE_4 in asthmatic subjects. Eur Resp J. 1994; 7: 907–13.

36. Westcott J, Sloan S, Wenzel S. Immunofiltration purification for urinary leukotriene quantification. Anal Biochem. 1997; 248: 202–10.

37. Dahlén B, Kumlin M, Margolskee DJ, et al. The leukotriene-receptor antagonist MK-0679 blocks airway obstruction induced by inhaled lysine-aspirin in aspirin-sensitive asthmatics. Eur Respir J. 1993; 6: 1018–26.

38. Kumlin M, Dahlén B. The challenge procedure influences the magnitude of allergen-induced urinary excretion of leukotriene E_4. Am J Resp Crit Care Med. 1997; 155: A665.

39. Dahlén B, Zetterström O. Comparison of bronchial and per oral provocation with aspirin in aspirin-sensitive asthmatics. Eur Resp J. 1990; 3: 527–34.

40. Granström E, Kumlin M, Kindahl H, Radioimmunoassay of eicosanoids. In: Benedetto C, McDonald-Gibson RG, Nigam S, Slater TF, editors. Prostaglandins and related substances: A practical approach. Oxford: IRL Press, 1987: 167–95.

41. Tagari P, Ethier D, Carry M, et al. Measurements of urinary leukotrienes by reverse-phase liquid chromatography and radioimmunoassay. Clin Chem. 1989; 35: 388–91.

42. Drazen JM, O'Brien J, Sparrow D, et al. Recovery of leukotriene E_4 from the urine of patients with airway obstruction. Am Rev Resp Dis. 1992; 146: 104–8.

43. Tsikas D, Fauler J, Gutzki FM, Röder Th, Bestmann HJ, Frölich JC. Gas chromatographic-mass spectrometric determination of leukotriene E_4 in human urine using deuterium-labelled leukotriene E_4 standards. J Chromatogr. 1993; 622: 1–7.

44. Nicoll-Griffith D, Zamboni R, Rasmussen JB, Ethier D, Charleson S, Tagari P. BIO-fully automated sample treatment high-performance liquid chromatography and radioimmunoassay for leukotriene E_4 in human urine from asthmatics. J Chromatogr. 1990; 526: 341–54.

45. Rasmussen JB, Eriksson L-O, Margolskee DJ, Tagari P, Williams VC, Andersson K-E. Leukotriene D_4 receptor blockade inhibits the immediate and late bronchoconstrictor responses to inhaled antigen in patients with asthma. J Allergy Clin Immunol. 1992; 90: 193–201.

46. Smith CM, Christie PE, Hawksworth RJ, Thien F, Lee TH. Urinary leukotriene E_4 levels after allergen and exercise challenge in bronchial asthma. Am Rev Resp Dis. 1991; 144: 1411–13.

47. Smith CM, Hawksworth RJ, Thien FCK, Christie PE, Lee TH. Urinary leukotriene E_4 in bronchial asthma. Eur Resp J. 1992; 5: 693–9.

48. Manning PJ, Rokach J, Malo J-L, et al. Urinary leukotriene E_4 levels during early and late asthmatic responses. J Allergy Clin Immunol. 1990; 86: 211–20.

49. Westcott JY, Smith HR, Wenzel SE, et al. Urinary leukotriene E_4 in patients with asthma. Effects of airways reactivity and sodium cromoglycate. Am Rev Resp Dis. 1991; 143: 1322–8.

50. Christie PE, Tagari P, Ford-Hutchinson AW, et al. Urinary leukotriene E_4 after lysine-aspirin inhalation in asthmatic subjects. Am Rev Resp Dis. 1992; 146: 1531–4.

51. Israel E, Rubin P, Kemp JP, et al. The effect of inhibition of 5-lipoxygenase by zileuton in mild-to-moderate asthma. Ann Intern Med. 1993; 119: 1059–66.

52. Taylor GW, Taylor I, Black P, et al. Urinary leukotriene E_4 after antigen challenge and in acute asthma and allergic rhinitis. Lancet. 1989; i: 584–8.

53. Sladek K, Dworski R, Fitzgerald GA, et al. Allergen-stimulated release of thromboxane A_2 and leukotriene E_4 in humans. Effects of indomethacin. Am Rev Resp Dis. 1990; 141: 1441–5.

54. Asano K, Lilly CM, O'Donell WJ, et al. Diurnal variation of urinary leukotriene E_4 and histamine excretion rates in normal subjects and patients with mild-to-moderate asthma. J Allergy Clin Immunol. 1995; 96: 643–51.

55. Bellia V, Bonanno A, Cibella F, et al. Urinary leukotriene E_4 in the assessment of nocturnal asthma. J Allergy Clin Immunol. 1996; 97: 735–41.

56. Wenzel SE, Trudeau JB, Kaminsky DA, Cohn J, Martin RJ, Westcott JY. Effect of 5-lipoxygenase inhibition on bronchoconstriction and airway inflammation in nocturnal asthma. Am J Resp Crit Care Med. 1995; 152: 897–905.

57. Szczeklik A. Aspirin-induced asthma: Pathogenesis and clinical presentation. Allergy Proc. 1992; 13: 163–73.

58. Christie PE, Tagari P, Ford-Hutchinson AW, et al. Urinary leukotriene E_4 concentrations

increase after aspirin challenge in aspirin-sensitive asthmatic subjects. Am Rev Resp Dis. 1991; 143: 1025–9.

59. Nasser SMS, Patel M, Bell GS, Lee TH. The effect of aspirin desensitization on urinary leukotriene E_4 concentrations in aspirin-sensitive asthma. Am J Resp Crit Care Med. 1995; 151: 1326–30.

60. Denzlinger C, Habert C, Wilmanns W. Cysteinyl leukotriene production in anaphylactic reactions. Int Arch Allergy Immunol. 1995; 108: 158–64.

61. Friedman BS, Bel EH, Buntinx A, et al. Oral leukotriene inhibitor (MK-886) blocks allergen-induced airway responses. Am Rev Resp Dis. 1993; 147: 839–44.

62. Hui KP, Taylor IK, Taylor GW, et al. Effect of a 5-lipoxygenase inhibitor on leukotriene generation and airway responses after allergen challenge in asthmatic patients. Thorax. 1991; 46: 184–9.

63. Nasser SMS, Bell GS, Hawksworth RJ, et al. Effect of the 5-lipoxygenase inhibitor ZD2138 on allergen-induced early and late asthmatic responses. Thorax. 1994; 49: 743–8.

64. Knapp HR, Sladek K, Fitzgerald GA. Increased excretion of leukotriene E_4 during aspirin-induced asthma. J Lab Clin Med. 1992; 119: 48–51.

65. Sladek K, Szczeklik A. Cysteinyl leukotrienes overproduction and mast cell activation in aspirin-provoked bronchospasm in asthma. Eur Resp J. 1993; 6: 391–9.

66. Nasser SMS, Bell GS, Foster S, et al. Effect of the 5-lipoxygenase inhibitor ZD2138 on aspirin-induced asthma. Thorax. 1994; 49: 749–56.

67. Sestini P, Armetti L, Gambaro G, et al. Inhaled PGE_2 prevents aspirin-induced bronchoconstriction and urinary LTE_4 excretion in aspirin-sensitive asthma. Am J Resp Crit Care Med. 1996; 153: 572–5.

68. Taylor IK, Wellings R, Taylor GW, Fuller RW. Urinary leukotriene E_4 excretion in exercise-induced asthma. J Appl Physiol. 1992; 73: 743–8.

69. Kikawa Y, Miyanomae T, Inoue Y, et al. Urinary leukotriene E_4 after exercise challenge in children with asthma. J Allergy Clin Immunol. 1992; 89: 1111–19.

70. Manning PJ, Watson RM, Margolskee DJ, Williams VC, Schwartz JI, O'Byrne PM. Inhibition of exercise-induced bronchoconstriction by MK-571: A potent leukotriene D_4-receptor antagonist. N Engl J Med. 1990; 323: 1736–9.

71. Finnerty JP, Wood-Baker R, Thomson H, Holgate ST. Role of leukotrienes in exercise-induced asthma. Inhibitory effect of ICI 204219, a potent leukotriene D_4 receptor antagonist. Am Rev Resp Dis. 1992; 145: 746–9.

72. Robuschi M, Riva E, Fucella LM, et al. Prevention of exercise-induced bronchoconstriction by a new leukotriene antagonist (SK&F 104353). A double-blind study versus disodium cromoglycate and placebo. Am Rev Resp Dis. 1992; 145: 1285–8.

73. Meltzer SS, Hasday JD, Cohn J, Bleecker ER. Inhibition of exercise-induced bronchospasm by zileuton: A 5-lipoxygenase inhibitor. Am J Resp Crit Care Med. 1996; 153: 931–5.

74. O'Sullivan S, Kumlin M, Larsson I, Roqut A, Dahlén B, Dahlén S-E. Urinary excretion of leukotriene E_4 and the mast cell marker $9\alpha,11\beta$-prostaglandin F_4 during allergen-induced early and late phase asthmatic reactions. Am J Resp Crit Care Med. 1996; 153: A250.

75. O'Sullivan S, Roquet A, Dahlén B, Kumlin M, Dahlén S-E. Urinary excretion of inflammatory mediators during allergen-induced early and late phase asthmatic reactions. Submitted.

76. Roquet A, Dahlén B, Kumlin M, et al. Combined antagonism of leukotrienes and histamine produces predominant inhibition of allergen-induced early and late phase airway obstruction in asthmatics. Am J Resp Crit Care Med. 1997; 155: 1856–63.

77. Taylor IK, O'Shaughnessy KM, Fuller RW, Dollery CT. Effect of cysteinyl-leukotriene receptor antagonist ICI 204,219 on allergen-induced bronchoconstriction and airway hyperreactivity in atopic subjects. Lancet. 1991; 337: 690–4.

78. Hansson G, Lindgren J, Dahlén S-E, Hedqvist P, Samuelsson B. Identification and biological activity of novel ω-oxidized metabolites of leukotriene B_4 from human leukocytes. FEBS Lett. 1981; 130: 107–12.

79. Schönfeld W, Schluter B, Hilger R, König W. Leukotriene generation and metabolism in isolated human lung macrophages. Immunology. 1988; 65: 529–36.

80. Kumlin M, Falck JR, Raud J, Harada Y, Dahlén S-E, Granström E. Identification and

biological activity of dihydro-leukotriene B_4: A prominent metabolite of leukotriene B_4 in the human lung. Biochem Biophys Res Commun. 1990; 170: 23–9.

81. Diamant Z, Timmers M, van der Veen H, et al. The effect of MK-0591, a novel 5-lipoxygenase activating protein inhibitor, on leukotriene biosynthesis and allergen-induced airway responses in asthmatic subjects in vivo. J Allergy Clin Immunol. 1995; 95: 42–51.

82. O'Sullivan S, Dahlén B, Dahlén S-E, Kumlin M. Increased urinary excretion of the prostaglandin D_2 metabolite $9\alpha,11\beta$-prostaglandin F_2 after aspirin challenge supports mast cell activation in aspirin-induced bronchoconstriction. J Allergy Clin Immunol. 1996; 98: 421–32.

83. Liston T, Roberts L. Metabolic fate of radiolabeled prostaglandin D_2 in a normal human male volunteer. J Biol Chem. 1985; 260: 13172–80.

84. Davidson D, Drafta D, Wilkens BA. Elevated urinary leukotriene E_4 in chronic lung disease of extreme prematurity. Am J Resp Crit Care Med. 1995; 151: 841–5.

85. Cook AJ, Yuksel B, Sampson AP, Greenough A, Price JF. Cysteinyl leukotriene involvement in chronic lung disease in premature infants. Eur Respir J. 1996; 9: 1907–12.

86. Fauler J, Neumann CH, Tsikas D, Frölich JC. Enhanced synthesis of cysteinyl leukotrienes in atopic dermatitis. Br J Dermatol. 1993; 128: 627–30.

87. Carry M, Korley V, Willerson JT, Weigelt L, Ford-Hutchinson AW, Tagari P. Increased urinary leukotriene excretion in patients with cardiac ischemia. In vivo evidence for 5-lipoxygenase activation. Circulation. 1992; 85: 230–6.

88. Allen SP, Sampson AP, Piper PJ, Chester AH, Ohri SK, Yacoub MH. Enhanced excretion of urinary leukotriene E_4 in coronary artery disease and after coronary artery bypass surgery. Coronary Artery Dis. 1993; 4: 899–904.

89. Fauler J, Thon A, Tsikas D, von der Hardt H, Frölich JC. Enhanced synthesis of cysteinyl leukotrienes in juvenile rheumatoid arthritis. Arthritis Rheum. 1994; 37: 93–7.

90. Hackshaw KV, Voelkel NF, Thomas RB, Westcott JY. Urine leukotriene E_4 levels are elevated in patients with active systemic lupus erythematosus. J Rheumatol. 1992; 19: 252–8.

91. Hackshaw KV, Yuhong SHI, Brandwein SR, Jones K, Westcott JY. A pilot study of zileuton, a novel selective 5-lipoxygenase inhibitor, in patients with systemic lupus erythematosus. J Rheumatol. 1995; 22: 462–8.

6 Influence of leukotrienes and anti-leukotrienes on airway tone and migration of inflammatory cells

B. E. A. LAMS and T. H. LEE

The leukotrienes (LTs) are generated by the enzyme 5-lipoxygenase (5-LO) which acts on arachidonic acid in conjunction with 5-LO activating protein (FLAP) to generate the unstable epoxide LTA_4 which is then either converted to LTB_4, or via LTC_4 synthase to the cysteinyl leukotriene (cys-LT) LTC_4. LTC_4 is converted by γ-glutamyltranspeptidase to LTD_4 and by a dipeptidase to LTE_4. The cysteinyl leukotrienes, LTC_4, LTD_4 and LTE_4, comprise the activity which was previously designated slow reacting substances of anaphylaxis.

There is increasing evidence that the cys-LTs play a role in the pathogenesis of bronchial asthma. Both in vitro and in vivo studies have shown that the LTs have an influence on airway tone, being important in causing bronchoconstriction and the induction of hyperresponsiveness. They also appear to affect infiltration of inflammatory cells. Studies on the recently developed LT antagonists and synthesis inhibitors have underlined the important role LTs play in airway tone in asthma.

BRONCHOCONSTRICTOR EFFECT OF THE LEUKOTRIENES

Isolated tracheal, bronchial or parenchymal tissues from guinea-pigs[1], dogs[2] and rats[3] contract in response to LTC_4 at nanomolar concentrations. In guinea-pig tissue, LTC_4 and LTD_4 are approximately equipotent as contractile agonists with EC_{50} values of 0.1 1 μM. LTE_4 is less potent in the same model with EC_{50} values of 30–100 nM[4,5]. In vitro studies on isolated human bronchus[6] and tracheal smooth muscle[7] have demonstrated a contractile action of LTC_4 with a potency 1000 times that of histamine.

In vivo studies have revealed a bronchoconstrictor effect of inhaled nebulized solutions of LTs in both normal and asthmatic individuals. In normal subjects, LTC_4 is 600–9500 times as potent as histamine in causing a 30% fall in expiratory flow at a lung volume of 30% of baseline vital capacity above residual volume[8]. LTD_4 is 6000 times more potent than histamine[9], while LTE_4 appears to be only 40–60 times as potent as histamine but has a longer duration of action than the other cys-LTs[10,11]. In asthmatic individuals, the LTs also have a bronchoconstrictor effect. However, in asthmatics LTC_4 is only 40 times as potent as histamine in inducing bronchoconstriction[12] and LTD_4 is only 140 times as potent[13]. Further studies have confirmed that the relative (to histamine) potencies of LTC_4 and LTD_4 are reduced in asthmatics compared with normal individuals[14].

A further study has shown that when compared to normal subjects, asthmatics have a 14-fold greater response to histamine, a 15-fold greater response to methacholine, a 6-fold greater response to LTC_4, a 9-fold greater response to LTD_4, and a 219-fold greater response to LTE_4. Furthermore, as airways became more hyper-responsive as judged by their response to histamine and methacholine, so the relative potency of LTE_4 increases when compared to LTC_4 and LTD_4[15]. Studies in asthmatics whose asthma is precipitated by aspirin have shown that these individuals are exquisitely sensitive to LTE_4 which is 1870 times more potent than histamine in aspirin-sensitive subjects and only 145 times more potent than histamine in asthmatics who are aspirin-tolerant[16].

INDUCTION OF HYPER-RESPONSIVENESS BY LTE$_4$

In addition to inducing contraction of guinea-pig smooth muscle, LTE_4 induces hyper-responsiveness to subsequent histamine administration in this tissue. Indomethacin, a cyclooxygenase inhibitor, inhibits this hyper-responsiveness but not the initial contraction suggesting that these two effects are mediated by different mechanisms[17]. The inhibition of hyper-responsiveness to histamine by indomethacin also implies that this may be mediated by prostanoids such as thromboxane A_2. Thromboxane A_2 is a potent agonist at the TP receptor and there is evidence that GR32191, a potent TP receptor antagonist blocks the histamine hyper-responsiveness induced by LTE_4[18]. This hyper-responsiveness is also inhibited by atropine and tetrodotoxin suggesting that cholinergic nerve transmission may play a role. It is possible that LTE_4 may induce hyper-responsiveness by the release of prostanoids, which then act on TP receptors located on cholinergic nerve terminals, thus priming these terminals to release increased amounts of acetylcholine when stimulated by histamine.

In vitro pretreatment of human bronchial smooth muscle with LTE_4 resulted in a four-fold decrease in histamine EC_{50} which was again inhibited by GR32191 and atropine, suggesting the involvement of the TP receptor and the muscarinic receptor as in guinea pig smooth muscle[18]. Arm et al.[19] have demonstrated that LTE_4 enhances histamine airway responsiveness in vivo in asthmatic subjects. This enhancement of airway responsiveness was significantly inhibited by indomethacin in a study of eight mildly asthmatic subjects[20], providing in vivo evidence that LTE_4-induced hyper-responsiveness to histamine is mediated in part by cyclooxygenase pathway-derived products.

Preincubation of epithelially denuded guinea-pig tracheal smooth muscle with LTE_4 in vitro increased the subsequent maximal response to histamine and substance P, suggesting that the response to epithelially intact tissues to both histamine and substance P after pretreatment with LTE_4 may be inhibited by an epithelium-derived factor[21].

EFFECTS ON MIGRATION OF INFLAMMATORY CELLS

In patients with bronchial asthma, instillation of LTE_4 followed by bronchial biopsy revealed an increase in eosinophils and neutrophils in the lamina propria. The selective recruitment of granulocytes but not of mononuclear cells suggests that cellular infiltration is unlikely to be caused by non specific leakage of cells from the circulation. Furthermore, the cellular influx was not seen after airflow obstruction provoked by methacholine challenge, suggesting that cellular influx was not due to bronchoconstriction per se[22].

When stimulated with LTC_4 and LTD_4, human endothelial cells in culture produce platelet activating factor (PAF), which remains associated with these cells[23]. LTC_4 and LTD_4 also induced the adherence of human neutrophils to the endothelial cell monolayer via an endothelial cell mediated process. The time course of neutrophil adhesion paralleled that of PAF production suggesting that PAF synthesized and retained by LTC_4- and LTD_4-stimulated endothelial cells may induce adherence of neutrophils. Thus, leukotrienes may be involved in the recruitment of inflammatory cells in addition to their effects on bronchoconstriction and induction of hyper-responsiveness.

ISOLATION OF LEUKOTRIENES FROM ASTHMATICS

Increased levels of LTC_4 and LTB_4[24] have been detected in bronchoalveolar lavage fluid (BALF) from asthmatic individuals at baseline. Other workers have found increased levels of LTC_4 in BALF after endobronchial allergen challenge[25]. Manning and others[26] found an increase in urinary LTE_4 in those with an early asthmatic response whereas those with an isolated late asthmatic response had no increase. Drazen and others[27] looked at 72 patients attending hospital emergency rooms with asthma and found that urinary LTE_4 levels were higher in those who responded to a nebulized bronchodilator when compared to those who did not, suggesting that cys-LTs may have a bronchospastic role in acute asthma. Christie and co-workers[28] demonstrated a 6-fold increase in urinary LTE_4 in aspirin-sensitive asthmatics compared with normal individuals and non-aspirin-sensitive asthmatics.

LEUKOTRIENE ANTAGONISTS

Several studies suggest that inhibition of LTD_4 action by LTD_4 ($CysLT_1$) receptor antagonists has a blunting effect on the fall in FEV_1 seen in asthmatics after experimental challenge with allergen, exercise, inhalation of cold dry air and aspirin. Ten asthmatics pretreated with the selective and potent second generation oral agent zafirlukast (ICI 204,219) showed a reduction of 80% in their early asthmatic response (EAR) and of 50% in their late asthmatic response (LAR) after allergen challenge[29]. Treatment also suppressed an increase in bronchial reactivity 6 h after challenge. The quinolone derivative MK571 has also been shown to inhibit the EAR by 88% and the LAR by 63%[30].

In a model of exercise-induced asthma, oral treatment with zafirlukast resulted in a reduction in the fall of FEV_1 after inhalation of cold dry air from 36% to 21% in eight asthmatics[31]. A further study on the same compound revealed a halving of the fall in FEV_1 after exercise in nine asthmatics[32]. MK571 also led to a 70% decrease in the fall in FEV_1 and a shortening in the recovery time from 33 minutes to 8 minutes in 12 asthmatics after exercise (Figure 1)[33].

Aspirin-sensitive asthma is probably the most LT dependent model for the investigation of anti-LT therapy. The weak LTD_4 antagonist pobilukast (SK&F 104,353) reduced

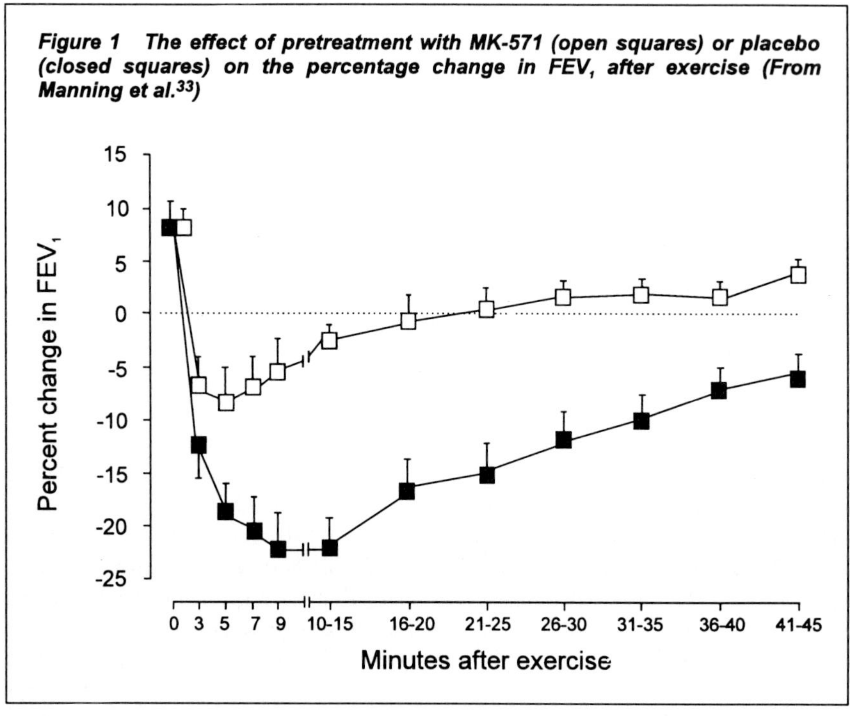

Figure 1 *The effect of pretreatment with MK-571 (open squares) or placebo (closed squares) on the percentage change in FEV₁ after exercise (From Manning et al.[33])*

the response to ingested aspirin by a mean of 47% in five out of six subjects[34]. The quinolone derivative MK679 (verlukast) improved baseline function in eight aspirin-sensitive asthmatics and blocked the airways obstruction caused by inhaled lysine aspirin, producing a 4.4-fold rightward shift in the dose–response curve[35].

Several studies have shown that LT antagonists have a bronchodilator effect on asthmatics. Intravenous treatment with MK679 led to an increase in baseline FEV_1 of up to 15.8% in nine asthmatics with resting FEV_1 of 40–80% of predicted[36]. Oral administration of zafirlukast led to an increase in resting FEV_1 compared with placebo, the effect of salbutamol being additive[37]. This additive effect was confirmed in a study of 12 asthmatics treated with intravenous MK571; the degree of bronchodilation was inversely proportional to the baseline FEV_1 and additive to that produced by albuterol[38].

LEUKOTRIENE BIOSYNTHESIS INHIBITORS

Studies using the 5-LO inhibitors (both direct and indirect, i.e. FLAP) have addressed their effect on the asthmatic response to challenge with allergen, cold air, exercise and aspirin. A study of the FLAP inhibitor MK886 revealed a 58% fall in the early asthmatic response of eight atopic men after allergen challenge and a fall in the late asthmatic response of 44%. This was accompanied by a 54% fall in A23187-stimulated whole blood LTB_4 generation, a 51.5% inhibition in the rise of urinary LTE_4 in the early asthmatic response and an 80% inhibition during the late asthmatic response[39].

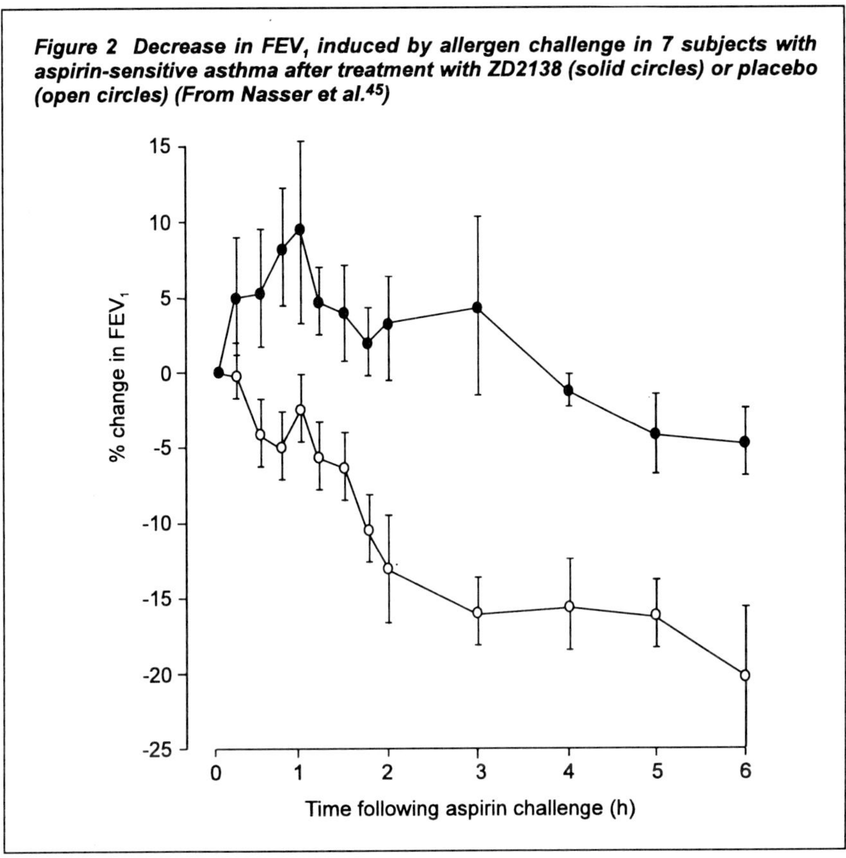

Figure 2 *Decrease in FEV₁ induced by allergen challenge in 7 subjects with aspirin-sensitive asthma after treatment with ZD2138 (solid circles) or placebo (open circles) (From Nasser et al.[45])*

Administration of the FLAP inhibitor MK0591 prior to allergen challenge led to a 96% inhibition of LTB_4 and an 84% inhibition of urinary LTE_4 production 24 h after allergen challenge. In addition there was a fall of 79% in the early asthmatic response and the late asthmatic response was delayed by 3 h[40]. BAYx1005, a FLAP inhibitor of similar potency to MK0591, was administered to atopic asthmatics and led to a reduction of 68% in the early asthmatic response to inhaled allergen and an 87% reduction in urinary LTE_4[41].

Thirteen asthmatics premedicated with a single dose of zileuton (a direct 5-LO inhibitor) had a reduction in ex vivo LTB_4 generation of 74% and an increase of 47% in the amount of cold air required to cause a fall in FEV_1 of 10%[42]. Zileuton pretreatment produced a 40% inhibition of bronchospasm post exercise with a reduction from 40 to 21 minutes in the time taken for FEV_1 to return to baseline values[43].

Treatment with zileuton in eight aspirin-sensitive asthmatics led to a fall in urinary LTE_4 of 70% and prevented a drop in FEV_1 after aspirin challenge[44]. Similarly, ZD2138 protects against aspirin-induced asthma with a 20.3% fall after challenge and treatment with placebo and a fall of 4.9% after treatment with ZD2138 associated with a reduction in whole blood LTB_4 generation of 72% and of urinary LTE_4 of 74% at 6 h (Figure 2)[45].

CONCLUSIONS

There is evidence from both in vitro and in vivo studies that the cys-LTs have an important influence on airway tone. These mediators have a potent bronchoconstrictor effect as well as inducing airway hyper-responsiveness. They also elicit the infiltration of inflammatory cells including eosinophils and neutrophils. Studies investigating LTD_4 receptor antagonism and 5-LO inhibition have provided compelling evidence for the importance of these mediators in the pathogenesis of asthma.

References

1. Piper PJ, Samhoun MN. The mechanism of action of leukotrienes C_4 and D_4 in guinea-pig isolated perfused lung and parenchymal strips of guinea pig, rabbit and rat. Prostaglandins. 1981; 21: 793–803.
2. Johnson HG, McNee ML. Secretogogue responses of leukotriene C_4, D_4: comparison of potency in canine trachea in vivo. Prostaglandins. 1983; 25: 237–43.
3. Szarek JL, Evans JN. Pharmacologic responsiveness of rat parenchymal strips, bronchi, and bronchioles. Exp Lung Res. 1988; 14: 575–85.
4. Dahlén S-E. Pulmonary effects of leukotrienes. Acta Physiol Scand Suppl. 1983; 512: 1–51.
5. Drazen JM, Austen KF. Leukotrienes and airway responses. Amer Rev Resp Dis. 1987; 136: 985–98.
6. Dahlén S-E, Hedqvist P, Hammarström S, Samuelsson B. Leukotrienes are potent constrictors of human bronchi. Nature. 1980; 288; 484–6.
7. Jones TR, Davis C, Daniel EE. Pharmacological study of the contractile activity of leukotriene C_4 and D_4 on isolated human airway smooth muscle. Can J Physiol Pharmacol. 1982; 60: 638–43.
8. Weiss JW, Drazen JM, Coles N, et al. Bronchoconstrictor effects of leukotriene C in humans. Science. 1982; 216: 196–8.
9. Weiss JW, Drazen JM, McFadden ER Jr, et al. Airway constriction in normal humans produced by inhalation of leukotriene D. Potency, time course, and effect of aspirin therapy. JAMA. 1983; 249: 2814–17.
10. Davidson AB, Lee TH, Scanlon PD, et al. Bronchoconstrictor effects of leukotriene E_4 in normal and asthmatic subjects. Amer Rev Resp Dis. 1987; 135: 333–7.
11. O'Hickey SP, Arm JP, Rees PJ, Spur BW, Lee TH. The relative responsiveness to inhaled leukotriene E_4, methacholine and histamine in normal and asthmatic subjects. Eur Resp J. 1988; 1: 913–7.
12. Smith LJ, Greenberger PA, Patterson R, Krell RD, Bernstein PR. The effect of inhaled leukotriene D_4 in humans. Amer Rev Res Dis. 1985; 131: 368–72.
13. Griffin M, Weiss JW, Leitch AG, et al. Effects of leukotriene D on the airways in asthma. New Engl J Med. 1983; 308: 436–9.
14. Barnes NC, Piper PJ, Costello JF. Actions of inhaled leukotrienes and their interactions with other allergic mediators. Prostaglandins. 1984; 28: 629–30.
15. Arm JP, O'Hickey SP, Hawksworth RJ, et al. Asthmatic airways have a disproportionate hyperresponsiveness to LTE_4, as compared with normal airways, but not to LTC_4, LTD_4, methacholine, and histamine. Amer Rev Resp Dis. 1990; 142: 1112–18.
16. Arm JP, O'Hickey SP, Spur BW, Lee TH. Airway responsiveness to histamine and leukotriene E_4 in subjects with aspirin-induced asthma. Amer Rev Resp Dis. 1989; 140: 148–53.
17. Lee TH, Austen KF, Corey EJ, Drazen JM. Leukotriene E_4-induced airway hyperresponsiveness of guinea pig tracheal smooth muscle to histamine and evidence for

three separate sulfidopeptide leukotriene receptors. Proc Natl Acad Sci USA. 1984; 81: 4922–5.

18. Jacques CA, Spur BW, Johnson M, Lee TH. Mechanism of LTE_4-induced histamine hyperresponsiveness in guinea-pig tracheal and human bronchial smooth muscle, in vitro. Br J Pharmacol. 1991; 104: 859–66.

19. Arm JP, Spur BW, Lee TH. The effects of inhaled leukotriene E_4 on the airway responsiveness to histamine in subjects with asthma and normal subjects. J Allergy Clin Immunol. 1988; 82: 654–60.

20. Christie PE, Hawksworth R, Spur BW, Lee TH. Effect of indomethacin on leukotriene$_4$ induced histamine hyperresponsiveness in asthmatic subjects. Amer Rev Resp Dis. 1992; 146: 1506–10.

21. Jacques CA, Spur BW, Johnson M, Lee TH. The effect of epithelium removal on leukotriene E_4-induced histamine hyperresponsiveness in guinea-pig tracheal smooth muscle. Brit J Pharmacol. 1992; 106: 556–62.

22. Laitinen LA, Laitinen A, Haahtela T, Lilkka V, Spur BW, Lee TH. Leukotriene E_4 and granulocytic infiltration into asthmatic airways. Lancet. 1993; 341: 989–90.

23. McIntyre TM, Zimmerman GA, Prescott SM. Leukotrienes C4 and D4 stimulate human endothelial cells to synthesize platelet activating factor and bind neutrophils. Proc Natl Acad Sci USA. 1986; 83: 2204–8.

24. Wardlaw AJ, Hay H, Cromwell O, Collins JV, Kay AB. Leukotrienes, LTC_4 and LTB_4, in bronchoalveolar lavage in bronchial asthma and other respiratory diseases. J Allergy Clin Immunol. 1989; 84: 19–26.

25. Wenzel SE, Larsen GL, Johnston K, Voelkel NF, Westcott JY. Elevated levels of leukotriene C_4 in bronchoalveolar lavage fluid from atopic asthmatics after endobronchial allergen challenge. Amer Rev Resp Dis. 1990; 142: 112–19.

26. Manning PJ, Rokach J, Malo JL, et al. Urinary leukotriene E_4 levels during early and late asthmatic responses. J Allergy Clin Immunol. 1990; 86: 211–20.

27. Drazen JM, O'Brien J, Sparrow D, Weiss ST, Martins MA, Israel E. Recovery of leukotriene E_4 from the urine of patients with airway obstruction. Am Rev Resp Dis. 1992; 146: 104–8.

28. Christie PE, Tagari P, Ford-Hutchinson AW, et al. Urinary leukotriene E_4 concentrations increase after aspirin challenge in aspirin-sensitive asthmatic subjects. Am Rev Resp Dis. 1991; 143: 1025–9.

29. Taylor IK, O'Shaughnessy KM, Fuller RW, Dollery CT. Effect of cysteinyl-leukotriene receptor antagonist ICI 204.219 on allergen-induced bronchoconstriction and airway hyperreactivity in atopic subjects. Lancet. 1991; 337: 690–4.

30. Rasmussen JB, Eriksson LO, Margolskee DJ, Tagari P, Williams VC. Leukotriene D_4 receptor blockade inhibits the immediate and late bronchoconstrictor responses to inhaled antigen in patients with asthma. J Allergy Clin Immunol. 1992; 90: 193–201.

31. Finnerty JP, Wood-Baker R, Thomson H, Holgate ST. Role of leukotrienes in exercise-induced asthma. Inhibitory effect of ICI 204,219, a potent leukotriene D_4 receptor antagonist. Am Rev Resp Dis. 1992; 145: 746–9.

32. Makker HK, Lau LC, Thomson HW, Binks SM, Holgate ST. The protective effect of inhaled leukotriene D_4 receptor antagonist ICI 204,219 against exercise-induced asthma. Am Rev Resp Dis. 1993; 147: 1413–18.

33. Manning PJ, Watson RM, Margolskee DJ, Williams VC, Schwartz JI. Inhibition of exercise-induced bronchoconstriction by MK-571, a potent leukotriene D_4-receptor antagonist [see comments]. N Engl J Med. 1990; 323: 1736–9.

34. Christie PE, Hawksworth R, Spur BW, Lee TH. Effect of indomethacin on leukotriene E_4-induced histamine hyperresponsiveness in asthmatic subjects. Am Rev Resp Dis. 1992; 146: 1506–10.

35. Dahlén B, Kumlin M, Margolskee DJ, et al. The leukotriene-receptor antagonist MK-0679 blocks airway obstruction induced by inhaled lysine-aspirin in aspirin-sensitive asthmatics. Eur Respir J. 1993; 6: 1018–26.

36. Impens N, Reiss TF, Teahan JA, et al. Acute bronchodilation with an intravenously administered leukotriene D_4 antagonist, MK-679. Am Rev Resp Dis. 1993; 147: 1442–6.

37. Hui KP, Barnes NC. Lung function improvement in asthma with a cysteinyl-leukotriene receptor antagonist. Lancet. 1991; 337: 1062–3.

38. Gaddy JN, Margolskee DJ, Bush RK, Williams VC, Busse WW. Bronchodilation with a potent and selective leukotriene D_4 (LTD_4) receptor antagonist (MK-571) in patients with asthma. Am Rev Resp Dis. 1992; 146: 358–63.

39. Friedman BS, Bel EH, Buntinx A, et al. Oral leukotriene inhibitor (MK-886) blocks allergen-induced airway responses. Am Rev Resp Dis. 1993; 147: 839–44.

40. Diamant Z, Timmers MC, van der Veen H, et al. The effect of MK-0591, a potent oral leukotriene biosynthesis inhibitor, on allergen-induced airway responses in asthmatic subjects. Eur Respir J. 1993; 6: 253.

41. Dahlén S-E, Dahlén B, Ihre E, et al. The leukotriene biosynthesis inhibitor BAYx1005 is a potent inhibitor of allergen-induced airway obstruction and leukotriene formation in man. Pulmon Pharmacol. 1993; 6: 87–96.

42. Israel E, Dermarkarian R, Rosenberg M, Sperling R, Taylor G, Rubin P. The effects of a 5-lipoxygenase inhibitor on asthma induced by cold, dry air. New Engl J Med. 1990; 323: 1740–4.

43. Meltzer SS, Rechsteiner EA, Johns MA, Cohn J, Bleecker ER. Inhibition of exercise-induced asthma by zileuton, a 5-lipoxygenase inhibitor. Am J Resp Crit Care Med. 1994; 149: A215.

44. Israel E, Fischer AR, Rosenberg MA, et al. The pivotal role of 5-lipoxygenase products in the reaction of aspirin-sensitive asthmatics to aspirin. Am Rev Resp Dis. 1993; 148: 1447–51.

45. Nasser SM, Bell GS, Foster S, et al. Effect of the 5-lipoxygenase inhibitor ZD2138 on aspirin-induced asthma. Thorax. 1994; 49: 749–56.

7 Leukotrienes in airways obstruction and inflammation evoked by allergen

N. C. BARNES and A. J. MACFARLANE

The first description of slow reacting substances (SRSs) was of their release from guinea-pig lung by cobra venom[1]. Shortly after this, it was shown that immunological challenge of guinea-pig lung resulted in the release of similar SRSs[2]. Since then the investigation of allergen challenge of sensitized tissues or whole animals has been central to the study of SRS-A and leukotrienes (LTs). Early studies into the biological actions of SRS-A suggested that it may be an important mediator in bronchial asthma. Later the structures of SRS-As derived from non-immunological and immunological challenges were elucidated and found to be a mixture of three cysteinyl LTs (cys-LTs), LTC_4, LTD_4 and LTE_4.

When exposed to challenge with aeroallergens, susceptible asthmatic subjects respond by developing one of two patterns of change in airway calibre. Most demonstrate an early asthmatic reaction (EAR), with bronchoconstriction developing within 10–15 minutes followed by spontaneous reversal within 1 h. Between 50 and 65% of subjects develop a second episode of airway narrowing 3–8 h later, the late asthmatic response (LAR). The LAR is characterized by associated tissue oedema[3], infiltration and activation of inflammatory cells such as eosinophils, lymphocytes and neutrophils[4] and increased bronchial hyperresponsiveness, and it is often used as a model of chronic asthma. In man, allergen challenge has been used to detect LT release in vivo[5,6]. For many of the drugs developed as 5-lipoxygenase (5-LO) inhibitors and LT receptor antagonists, initial studies into their efficacy involve the study of antigen challenge and assessment of their effect on the EAR and LAR.

RESPONSES OF ISOLATED LUNG TISSUE TO ALLERGEN CHALLENGE

When isolated lung tissue of guinea pigs or rats sensitized to ovalbumin is challenged with ovalbumin it contracts. This contraction can be partially attenuated by histamine (H_1) receptor antagonists, but a residual contraction of slow onset and prolonged duration remains[7]. Biological assays of the effluent fluid released by allergen challenge of perfused or minced lung tissues from a variety of sensitized animals demonstrated the release of SRS-A, which provoked a more prolonged contraction of guinea-pig ileum than that induced by histamine alone[2]. When the effects of histamine were blocked by an H_1 antagonist the activity of SRS-A remained[8].

Improved analytical techniques such as high pressure liquid chromatography (HPLC)[9] and radioimmunoassays (RIAs) for cys-LTs[10] demonstrated that the major non-histamine bronchoconstrictor substances released from sensitized guinea-pig and rat lung were LTs[9,11,12]. Using human lung tissue, obtained after surgical resection from asthmatic patients, Dahlén et al. were able to demonstrate cys-LT formation in response to specific allergen challenge[13]. They went on to demonstrate the release of LTs from lung tissue obtained after surgical resection from non-asthmatic, non-atopic subjects, in response to allergen exposure following passive sensitization[14].

The effect of anti-asthmatic drugs on LT release has been studied. As glucocorticosteroids are known to inhibit the LAR provoked by allergen[15] interest focused on their effect on LT synthesis. It is possible to show that glucocorticosteroids inhibit formation of LTs and other eicosanoids in vitro[16,17] but only at significantly higher concentrations than those obtained in vivo. At the inhaled or systemic steroid concentrations that are used in asthma it has proved difficult to inhibit LT synthesis in man[17,18].

Investigations into the effect of LT receptor antagonists and 5-LO inhibitors often involve the investigation of their effects on allergen responses in sensitized lung tissue. LT receptor antagonists markedly attenuate antigen-induced airway smooth muscle contraction in both guinea-pig tracheal rings and human bronchial strips[7]. When combined with a histamine receptor antagonist, both LT receptor antagonists and 5-LO inhibitors prevent antigen-induced bronchospasm in these models[7,19].

ALLERGEN-INDUCED RESPONSES IN WHOLE ANIMAL MODELS

Allergen-induced bronchospasm in whole animal models has also been used to investigate the role of LTs in allergic responses akin to allergen-induced bronchoconstriction in man. The most commonly studied animal model is the guinea pig, but there has also been a substantial amount of work performed on the allergic sheep model and some interesting work in *Ascaris*-sensitive squirrel monkeys[20,21].

Allergen challenge of sensitized guinea pigs results in anaphylactic reaction caused by massive histamine release[22]. Pretreatment with an H_1 antagonist enables them to survive and reveals an EAR[22]. This response can be largely abolished with LT receptor antagonists or 5-LO inhibitors[19,22,23]. Although the LAR is less easy to study, it has also been shown to be attenuated by drugs acting against the LT pathway[23].

Sheep naturally sensitized to *Ascaris suum* offer a well characterized model, demonstrating a reproducible EAR and LAR to inhaled allergen[24]. Following allergen challenge, LTs are released into the airways of these sheep using bronchoalveolar lavage (BAL)[24,25]. Inhalation of LTD_4 in this model will also provide a biphasic bronchoconstrictor response with clear early and late phases[26], both of which can be attenuated by LT receptor antagonists and 5-LO inhibitors[27,28].

LEUKOTRIENE RELEASE IN MAN

Increased levels of LTs have been demonstrated in nasal washings of patients sensitive to ragweed after intranasal allergen challenge[29]. Non-allergic subjects challenged with intranasal ragweed pollen developed neither symptoms nor LT release[29]. The rise in

LT levels in nasal lavage fluid is biphasic, suggesting that LT synthesis occurs during both the early and the late phase response[30].

Using the technique of BAL following allergen challenge, increased levels of cys-LTs and LTB_4 can be collected from asthmatic patients[3,5,6,31]. However it has proved very difficult to measure LT levels in blood in man. This is thought to be due to the low levels of LTs present and to the presence of other substances which cross-react with the RIA[32]. As there is a limit to the number of bronchoscopies that can be performed in an asthmatic patient it is not possible to perform serial BAL to monitor the LT synthesis during the EAR and LAR.

The demonstration that 4–6% of all LT synthesized appears in the urine as LTE_4 has proved extremely useful, enabling the evaluation of LT synthesis following allergen challenge[33–35]. Taylor et al. studied urinary LTE_4 levels in asthmatic patients and clearly demonstrated a rise in LTE_4 during the EAR[33]. Similar results were found by other groups, who demonstrated a rise in LTE_4 levels during the EAR but not the LAR[34,36]. It was, therefore, unexpected when LT antagonists were shown to have a marked effect on blocking the LAR. This apparent contradiction has been resolved by recent studies using more accurate urine analysis techniques and carefully timed collections to show that urinary LTE_4 levels are also raised during the LAR[37]. This study also demonstrated that both the early and the late rise in urinary LTE_4 could be inhibited by the 5-LO activating protein (FLAP) inhibitor MK-0591 (Figure 1)[37].

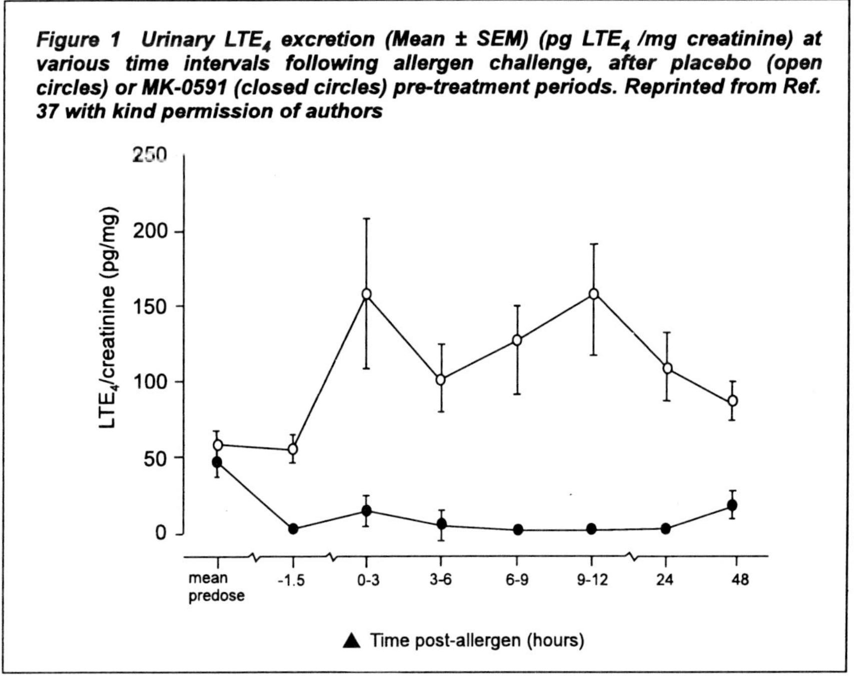

Figure 1 Urinary LTE_4 excretion (Mean ± SEM) (pg LTE_4/mg creatinine) at various time intervals following allergen challenge, after placebo (open circles) or MK-0591 (closed circles) pre-treatment periods. Reprinted from Ref. 37 with kind permission of authors

INVESTIGATION OF LEUKOTRIENE RECEPTOR ANTAGONISTS AND 5-LIPOXYGENASE INHIBITORS

The first LT antagonist was synthesized and described before the structure of SRS-A was elucidated[38]. FPL-55712 was able to block allergen-induced responses in isolated guinea-pig lung tissue[7] and was subject to a limited number of studies in man[7,39]. For example, FPL-55712 was shown to attenuate the normal decrease in mucociliary clearance occurring after allergen challenge[39] and close examination of the data also suggests it produced an effect on lung function. Thus, even with this early weak LT antagonist, with a very short half life, there was evidence of an effect on allergen-induced responses.

One of the next drugs studied was piriprost (U-60,257). In vitro it blocked production of LTs[40] and eliminated contraction of asthmatic bronchi following allergen challenge[40]. Results of a double-blind, placebo-controlled study, showing no effect on the EAR were, therefore, disappointing[41]. Unfortunately no effort was made to confirm inhibition of LT synthesis. A similar study using the 5-LO inhibitor, nafazatrom showed the same lack of effect on the EAR. However in this study, evidence for 5-LO inhibition in vivo was sought and found to be lacking[42].

The first LT antagonists to unequivocally show activity in allergen challenge were the acetophenones L-649,923[43,44] and LY-171,883[27,45]. These both cause a small (3 to 10-fold) shift to the right in the dose–response curve to inhaled LTD_4[44,45] and cause a small but statistically significant attenuation of the EAR, but not the LAR[27,43,46]. Thus it seemed that either the LTs were not important mediators of allergic responses or that even these weak antagonists of these important mediators could produce an effect.

When the second generation of LT receptor antagonists such as ICI-204,219 (zafirlukast), MK-571, ONO-1078 (pranlukast) and montelukast[47] were studied full appreciation of the role of LTs became possible. These are potent LT antagonists, capable of shifting the dose–response curve to inhaled LTD_4 up to 100-fold to the right[48–50].

A single oral dose of zafirlukast (40 mg) given before challenge blocks approximately 70% of the EAR to inhaled allergen and 50% of the LAR[51] (see Figure 2). In addition, it attenuates the bronchial hyper-responsiveness seen after challenge. However, as these measurements were taken at 6 h, when the patients still demonstrated a degree of bronchoconstriction, the relevance of this observation is not clear[52]. Similar results have been obtained with the other LT receptor antagonists such as MK-571[53] and biosynthesis inhibitors such as MK-886[54]. It now appears that the majority of the EAR is due to LTs with a small contribution from histamine, while LTs are responsible for approximately 50% of the bronchoconstriction in the LAR. It is probable that the effect on the EAR is purely to block airway smooth muscle contraction caused by LTs[43,46]. The LAR is thought to be due to a combination of cellular influx, tissue oedema and smooth muscle spasm. Whether LT antagonists are acting on the airway smooth muscle spasm, the cellular infiltrate, oedema formation or some combination of these processes is not yet clear and is the subject of current interest.

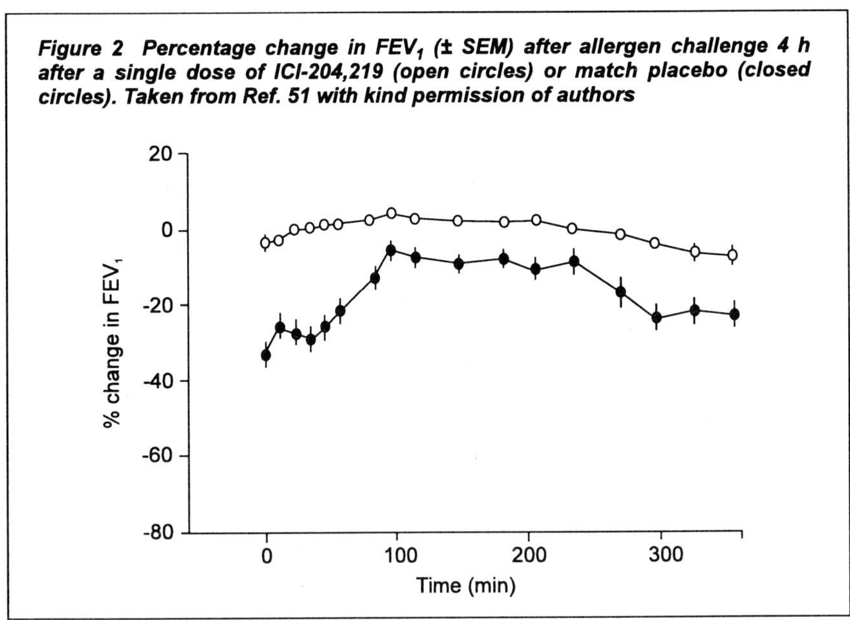

Figure 2   Percentage change in FEV$_1$ (± SEM) after allergen challenge 4 h after a single dose of ICI-204,219 (open circles) or match placebo (closed circles). Taken from Ref. 51 with kind permission of authors

The effect of drugs blocking LT production on the response to antigen challenge has been less impressive than the effects of antagonists. At a single dose of 800 mg, the direct 5-LO inhibitor zileuton produced only a non-significant attenuation of the EAR and had no effect on the LAR[55]. This was despite having a marked effect on LTB$_4$ production in ex vivo calcium ionophore-stimulated whole blood and blocking 50% of the urinary production of LTE$_4$[55]. This study also showed a correlation between blockade of urinary LTE$_4$ production and the attenuation of the EAR. Despite this rather poor effect on allergen challenge, zileuton has been shown to be of clinical benefit in asthma[56]: a single dose of 600 mg can improve lung function acutely in wheezy, bronchoconstricted asthmatics[56]. This discrepancy may be explained by the need for chronic treatment with zileuton prior to antigen challenge or to the exposures being performed too long after dosing resulting in inadequate 5-LO inhibition.

The FLAP antagonist MK-591 has a significant effect on the EAR (70% inhibition) but only a modest inhibition of the LAR[57]. The FLAP inhibitor BAYx1005 can also be shown to attenuate the EAR and LAR to allergen challenge, the magnitude of the blockade being similar to that seen with the potent LT receptor antagonists[58].

INFLAMMATORY CELL RESPONSES TO INHALED ALLERGEN

One question that remains to be answered completely is whether LTs actually have an effect on cellular infiltration. This is an important question since it may determine whether or not the drugs which modulate the actions of LTs can be expected to have an anti-inflammatory role in asthma. Initially it was thought that LTB$_4$ may prove to be an important pro-inflammatory mediator in asthma. Its actions include potent neutrophil chemotaxis, weak chemotactic and chemokinetic activity for eosinophils[59,60] as well as activation of neutrophils[61] and increasing their adherence to endothelial cells[62]. However evidence is mounting to suggest that LTB_4 may not contribute significantly to chronic asthma. Inhalation of LTB_4 results in neither changes in airway calibre nor increased bronchial hyper-responsiveness[63]. The effects of the LTB_4 receptor antagonist LY-293,111 on inhaled allergen challenge have been studied[64]. Although 7 days' pretreatment with LY-293,111 caused a profound reduction in neutrophil influx and activation status in the BAL 24 h following allergen challenge, there was no effect on eosinophil recruitment[64]. There was also no effect on either the EAR or LAR.

Animal models suggest that cys-LTs are important in the accumulation of eosinophils into both lungs of guinea-pigs[65,66] and primates. In one such study zafirlukast inhibited bronchial hyper-responsiveness and influx of eosinophils into the BAL fluid of cynomolgus monkeys following allergen challenge when compared with placebo[67].

Preliminary results of two segmental allergen challenges after zafirlukast or placebo in humans have been reported. Treatment for one week at a dose of 20 mg b.d. was shown to cause a decrease in influx of lymphocytes and basophils in the lavage fluid and a decrease in activation of alveolar macrophages 48 h after challenge[68]. At the higher dose of 160 mg twice daily the reduction in the number of basophils and activation status of macrophages was confirmed. There was also a significant reduction in the influx of eosinophils into the lavage fluid in this study[69]. These results suggest that LTs not only play a role as smooth muscle spasmogens but also cause inflammatory cell accumulation and activation after antigen challenge.

CONCLUSIONS

Allergen-induced responses have provided invaluable information at all stages in the understanding of LT biology. Future work to complete our understanding of the role of LTs in asthma will no doubt continue to rely on the study of antigen-induced responses and assessment of how their actions may be modified using potent and specific LT receptor antagonists and synthesis inhibitors.

Acknowledgement

We are grateful to *The Lancet* for permission to reproduce Figure 2 from reference 51 and to the *Journal of Allergy and Clinical Immunology* for permission to reproduce figure 1 from reference 37.

References

1. Feldberg W, Kellaway CH. Liberation of histamine from the perfused lung by snake venom. J Physiol. 1937; 90: 257–79.
2. Kellaway CH, Trethewie ER. The liberation of a slow-reacting smooth muscle stimulating substance in anaphylaxis. Q J Exp Physiol. 1940; 30: 121–45.

3. Diaz P, Gonzalez MC, Galleguillos FR, et al. Leukocytes and mediators in bronchoalveolar lavage during allergen-induced late phase asthmatic reactions. Am Rev Resp Dis. 1989; 139: 1383–9.

4. Cartier A, Thomson NC, Frith PA, Roberts R, Hargreave FE. Allergen-induced increase in bronchial responsiveness to histamine; relationship to the late asthmatic response and change in airway calibre. J Allergy Clin Immunol. 1982; 70: 170–7.

5. Miadonna A, Tedeschi A, Brasca C, Folco G, Sala A, Murphy RC. Mediator release after endobronchial antigen challenge in patients with respiratory allergy. J Allergy Clin Immunol. 1990; 85: 906–13.

6. Wenzel SE, Larsen GL, Johnston K, Voelkel NF, Westcott JY. Elevated levels of leukotriene C4 in bronchoalveolar lavage fluid from atopic asthmatics after endobronchial allergen challenge. Am Rev Resp Dis. 1990; 142: 112–19.

7. Adams GK, Lichtenstein L. In vitro studies of antigen-induced bronchospasm: Effect of antihistamine and SRS-A antagonist on response of sensitized guinea-pig and human airways to allergen. J Immunol. 1979; 122: 555–62.

8. Brocklehurst WE. The release of histamine and formation of a slow reacting substance (SRS-A) during anaphylactic shock. J Physiol. 1960; 151: 416–35.

9. Morris HR, Taylor GW, Piper PJ, Sirois P, Tippins JR. Slow reacting substance of anaphylaxis: Purification and characterisation. FEBS Lett. 1978; 87: 203–6.

10. Beaubien BC, Tippins JR, Morris HR. Leukotriene biosynthesis and metabolism detected by the combined use of HPLC and radioimmunoassay. Biochem Biophys Res Commun. 1984; 125: 97–104.

11. Morris HR, Piper PJ, Taylor GW, Tippins JR. Comparative studies on immunologically and non-immunologically produced slow reacting substances from man, guinea-pig and rat. Br J Pharmacol. 1979; 67: 179–84.

12. Brunet G, Charleson S, Ford-Hutchinson AW. Antigen-induced leukotriene release from rat lungs in vitro. Prostaglandins. 1985; 29: 921–32.

13. Dahlén SE, Hasson G, Hedquist P, Bjork T, Granstrom E, Dahlén B. Allergen challenge of lung tissue from asthmatics elicits bronchial contraction that correlates with the release of leukotrienes C4, D4, and E4. Proc Natl Acad Sci USA. 1983; 80: 1712–18.

14. Kumlin M, Dahlén SE. Leukotriene release in chopped human lung: Characteristics and regulation. Agents Actions. 1989; 26: 84–6.

15. Delehunt JC, Yerger L, Ahmed T, Abraham WM. Inhibition of antigen-induced bronchoconstriction by methyl prednisolone succinate. J Allergy Clin Immunol. 1984; 57: 1182–8.

16. Schleimer RP, Schulman ES, MacGlashan DW, et al. Effects of dexamethasone on mediator release from human lung fragments and purified lung mast cells. J Clin Invest. 1983; 71: 1830–5.

17. Sebaldt RJ, Sheller JA, Oates JA, Roberts LJ, FitzGerald GA. Inhibition of eicosanoid biosynthesis by glucocorticosteroids in humans. Proc Natl Acad Sci USA. 1990; 87: 6974–8.

18. Manso G, Baker AJ, Taylor IK, Fuller RW. In vivo and in vitro effects of glucocorticosteroids on arachidonic acid metabolism and monocyte function in non-asthmatic humans. Eur Resp J. 1992; 5: 712–16.

19. Malo PE, Bell RL, Shaughnessy TK, Summers JB, Brooks DW, Carter GW. The 5-lipoxygenase inhibitory activity of zileuton in vitro and in vivo models of antigen-induced airway anaphylaxis. Pulm Pharmacol. 1994; 7: 73–9.

20. Hamel R, McFarlane CS, Ford-Hutchinson AW. Late pulmonary responses induced by *Ascaris* allergen in conscious squirrel monkeys. J Appl Physiol. 1986; 61: 2081–7.

21. McFarlane CS, Hamel R, Ford-Hutchinson AW. Effects of a 5-lipoxygenase inhibitor (L-651,392) on primary and late pulmonary responses to *Ascaris* antigen in the squirrel monkey. Agents Actions. 1987; 22: 63–8.

22. Daffonchio L, Lees IW, Payne AW, White BJ. Pharmacological modulation of anaphylaxis induced by aerosol challenge in anaesthetised guinea-pigs. Br J Pharmacol. 1987; 91: 701–8.

23. Howell RE, Sickels BD, Woeppel SL, Jenkins LP, Rubin EB, Weichman BM. Leukotrienes mediate antigen-induced airway hyper-reactivity in guinea-pigs. J Pharmacol Exp Ther. 1994; 268: 353–8.

24. Abraham WM, Delehunt JC, Yerger L, Marchette B. Characterisation of a late phase

pulmonary response following antigen challenge in allergic sheep. Am Rev Resp Dis. 1983; 128: 839–44.

25. Okayama H, Aikawa T, Ontsu H, Sasaki H, Takishima T. Leukotriene C4 and B4 in bronchoalveolar lavage fluid during biphasic allergic bronchoconstriction in sheep. Am Rev Resp Dis. 1989; 139: 725–31.

26. Abraham WM, Russi E, Wanner A, Delehunt JC, Yerger LD, Chapman GA. Production of early and late pulmonary responses with inhaled leukotriene LTD4 in allergic sheep. Prostaglandins. 1985; 29: 715–27.

27. Abraham WM, Wanner A, Stevenson JS, Chapman AG. The effects of orally active leukotriene D4/E4 antagonist LY-171,883 on antigen-induced airway responses in allergic sheep. Prostaglandins. 1988; 3: 457–67.

28. Abraham WM, Stevenson JS, Garrido. A leukotriene and thromboxane inhibitor (Sch37224) blocks antigen-induced immediate and late responses and airway hyper-responsiveness in allergic sheep. J Pharm Exp Ther. 1988; 247: 1004–11.

29. Creticos PS, Peters SP, Adkinson NF, et al. Peptide leukotriene release after antigen challenge in patients sensitive to ragweed. N Engl J Med. 1986; 315: 800–4.

30. Naclerio RM, Baroody FM, Togias AG. The role of leukotrienes in allergic rhinitis: A review. Am Rev Resp Dis. 1991; 143: S91–5.

31. Wenzel SE, Westcott JY, Larsen GL. Bronchoalveolar lavage fluid mediator levels 5 minutes after allergen challenge in atopic subjects with asthma: Relationship to the development of late asthmatic responses. J Allergy Clin Immunol. 1991; 87: 540–8.

32. Heavy DJ, Soberman RJ, Lewis RA, Spur B, Austen KF. Critical considerations in the development of an assay for sulfidopeptide leukotrienes in the plasma. Prostaglandins. 1987; 33: 693–708.

33. Taylor G, Taylor I, Black P, et al. Urinary leukotriene E4 after antigen challenge and in acute asthma and allergic rhinitis. Lancet. 1989; 1: 584–8.

34. Kumlin M, Dahlén B, Bjorck T, et al. Urinary excretion of leukotriene E4 and 11-dehydro-thromboxane B2 in response to bronchial provocation with allergen, aspirin, leukotriene D4 and histamine in asthmatics. Am Rev Resp Dis. 1992; 146: 96–103.

35. Christie PE, Tagari P, Ford-Hutchinson SW, et al. Increased urinary LTE4 excretion following inhalation of LTC4 and LTE4 in asthmatic subjects. Eur Resp J. 1994; 7: 907–13.

36. Manning PJ, Rokach J, Malo J-L, et al. Urinary leukotriene E4 levels during early and late asthmatic responses. J Allergy Clin Immunol. 1990; 86: 211–20.

37. Diamant Z, Timmers MC, Van der Veen H, et al. The effect of MK-0591, a novel 5-lipoxygenase activating protein (FLAP) inhibitor, on leukotriene biosynthesis and allergen-induced airway responses in asthmatic subjects in vivo. J Allergy Clin Immunol. 1995; 1: 42–51.

38. Augstein J, Farmer JB, Lee TB, Sheard P, Tattersal ML. Selective inhibitor of slow reacting substance of anaphylaxis. Nature. 1973; 245: 215–17.

39. Ahmed T, Greenblatt D, Birch S, Marchette B, Wanner A. Abnormal mucociliary transport in allergic patients with antigen-induced bronchospasm: Role of slow reacting substance of anaphylaxis. Am Rev Resp Dis. 1981; 124: 110–14.

40. Bach MK, Brashler JR, Smith HW, Fitzpatrick FA, Sun FF, McGuire JC. 6,9-deepoxy-6,9-(phenylimino)-delta 6,8-prostaglandin I_1 (U-60,257), a new inhibitor of leukotriene C and D synthesis: In vitro studies. Prostaglandins. 1982; 23: 759–71.

41. Mann JS, Robinson C, Sheridan A, Clement P, Back MK, Holgate ST. Effect of inhaled Piriprost (U-60,257) a novel leukotriene inhibitor, on allergen and exercise induced bronchoconstriction in asthma. Thorax. 1986; 41: 746–52.

42. Fuller RW, Maltby N, Richmond R, et al. Oral Nafazatrom in man: Effect on inhaled antigen challenge. Br J Clin Pharmacol. 1987; 23: 677–81.

43. Britton JR, Hanley SP, Tattersfield AE. The effect of an oral leukotriene D4 antagonist L-649,923 on the response to inhaled antigen in asthma. J Allergy Clin Immunol. 1987; 79: 811–16.

44. Barnes NC, Piper PJ, Costello J. The effect of an oral leukotriene antagonist L-649,923 on histamine and leukotriene D4 induced bronchoconstriction in normal man. J Allergy Clin Immunol. 1987; 79: 816–21.

45. Phillips GD, Rafferty P, Robinson C, Holgate S. Dose-related antagonism of leukotriene

D4 induced bronchoconstriction by p.o. administration of LY-171,883 in non asthmatic subjects. J Pharmacol Exp Ther. 1988; 246: 732–8.

46. Fuller RW, Black PN, Dollery CT. Effect of the oral leukotriene D4 antagonist LY-171,883 on inhaled and intradermal challenge with antigen and LTD4 in atopic subjects. J Allergy Clin Immunol. 1989; 83: 939–44.

47. Jones TR, Labelle M, Belley M, et al. Pharmacology of montelukast sodium (singulair), a potent and selective leukotriene D4 receptor antagonist. Can J Physiol Pharmacol. 1995; 73: 191–201.

48. Smith LJ, Geller S, Elbright L, et al. Inhibition of leukotriene D4-induced bronchoconstriction in the human. Am Rev Resp Dis. 1990; 141: 988–92.

49. Kips JC, Joos GF, de Lepeleire I, et al. MK-571, a potent antagonist of leukotriene D4-induced bronchoconstriction in the human. Am Rev Resp Dis. 1991; 144: 617–21.

50. O'Shaughnessy TC, Georgiou P, Howland K, Barnes NC. The effect of pranlukast, an oral leukotriene antagonist, on leukotriene D_4 (LTD4) challenge in normal male subjects. Am J Resp Crit Care Med. 1995; 151: A378.

51. Taylor IK, O'Shaughnessy KM, Fuller RW, Dollery CT. Effect of cysteinyl-leukotriene receptor antagonist ICI-204,219 on allergen-induced bronchoconstriction and airway hyper-reactivity in atopic subjects. Lancet. 1991; 337: 690–4.

52. Aalbers R, de Monchy JG. Cysteinyl-leukotriene receptor antagonist, bronchoconstriction and airway hyperreactivity. Lancet. 1991; 338: 445.

53. Rasmussen JB, Eriksson LO, Margolskee DJ, et al. Leukotriene D_4 receptor blockade inhibits the immediate and late bronchoconstrictor responses to inhaled antigen in patients with asthma. J Allergy Clin Immunol. 1992; 90: 193–201.

54. Friedman BS, Bel EH, Buntinx A, et al. Oral leukotriene inhibitor (MK-886) blocks allergen-induced airway responses. Am Rev Resp Dis. 1993; 147: 839–44.

55. Hui KP, Taylor IK, Taylor GW, et al. Effect of a 5-lipoxygenase inhibitor on leukotriene generation and airway responses after allergen challenge in asthmatic patients. Thorax. 1991; 46: 184–9.

56. Israel E, Rubin P, Kemp JP, et al. The effect of inhibition of 5-lipoxygenase by Zileuton in mild to moderate asthma. Am Intern Med. 1993; 119: 1059–66.

57. Diamant Z, Timmers MC, Van der Veen H, et al. The effect of MK-591, a potent oral leukotriene biosynthesis inhibitor, on allergen-induced airway responses in asthmatic subjects. Eur Resp J. 1993; 6: 253.

58. Gardiner PJ, Cuthbert NJ, Francis HP, et al. Inhibition of antigen-induced contraction of guinea-pig airways by a leukotriene synthesis inhibitor BAY-x-1005. Eur J Pharm. 1994; 258: 95–102.

59. Palmer RMJ, Stepney RJ, Higgs GA, Eakins KE. Chemokinetic activity of arachidonic acid lipoxygenase products on leukocytes of different species. Prostaglandins. 1980; 20: 411–18.

60. Nagy L, Lee TH, Goetzl EJ, Pickett WC, Kay AB. Complement receptor enhancement and chemotaxis of human neutrophils and eosinophils by leukotrienes and other lipoxygenase products. Clin Exp Immunol. 1982; 47: 541–7.

61. Goldman DW, Goetzl EJ. Selective transduction of human polymorphonuclear leukocyte functions by subsets of receptors for leukotriene B_4. J Allergy Clin Immunol. 1984; 74: 373–7.

62. Hoover RL, Karnovsky MJ, Austen KF, Corey EJ, Lewis RA. Leukotriene B_4 action of endothelium mediates augmented neutrophil/endothelial adhesion. Proc Natl Acad Sci USA. 1984; 81: 2191–3.

63. Black PN, Fuller RW, Taylor GW, Barnes PJ, Dollery CT. Effect of inhaled leukotriene B_4 alone and in combination with prostaglandin D2 on bronchial responsiveness to histamine in normal subjects. Thorax. 1989; 44: 491–5.

64. Evans DJ, Barnes PJ, Spaethe SM, Van Alstyne EL, Mitchell MI, O'Conner BJ. The effect of a leukotriene B_4 receptor antagonist, LY-293,111, on allergen-induced responses in asthma. Thorax. 1996; 51: 1178–84.

65. Underwood DC, Osborn RR, Bochonwicz S, Newsholme SJ, Torphy TJ, Hay DWP.

Pranlukast, a potent and selective cysteinyl-leukotriene (CysLT) receptor antagonist, attenuates pro-inflammatory responses induced by leukotriene (LT) D_4. Eur Resp J. 1996; 9 (Suppl. 23): 288s.

66. Underwood DC, Osborn RR, Newsholme SJ, Torphy TJ, Hay DWP. Persistant airway eosinophilia after leukotriene D_4 administration in conscious guinea-pigs: Modulation by a peptidoleukotriene antagonist and interleukin (IL-5) monoclonal antibody. Asthma, Theory to Treatment. 1995 July 15–17 (abstract).

67. Turner CR, Smith WB, Andresen CJ, Swindell AC, Watson JW. Leukotriene D_4 receptor antagonism reduces airway hyperresponsiveness in monkeys. Pulm Pharmacol. 1994; 7: 49–58.

68. Calhoun WJ, Lavins BJ, Glass M. Effect of Accolate (zafirlukast) on bronchoalveolar lavage fluid (BAL) after segmental antigen bronchoprovocation (SBP) in patients with mild to moderate asthma. Am J Resp Crit Care Med. 1995; 151: A42.

69. Calhoun WJ, Williams KL, Simonson SG and Lavins BJ. Effect of zafirlukast (Accolate) on airway inflammation after segmental allergen challenge in patients with mild asthma. Am J Resp Crit Care Med. 1997; 155: A662.

8 Leukotrienes in induced airway obstruction

K. F. RABE

Under in vitro conditions, human isolated airways from non-atopic individuals exhibit inherent smooth muscle tone which is believed to be mainly the result of a balance of contractile cysteinyl-leukotrienes (cys-LTs), and, to a lesser extent, histamine[1] and bronchodilator prostanoids, such as prostaglandin E_2. While the source of the prostanoid is believed to be airway epithelial cells[2], histamine and leukotrienes (LTs) are likely to be produced by resident mast cells in the airway wall[3]. The role and physiological relevance of cys-LTs in airway tone in vivo is demonstrated by a series of clinical studies which showed that leukotriene-modifying drugs such as 5-lipoxygenase (5-LO) inhibitors[4] and cys-LT antagonists affect lung function after chronic dosing[5–10], irrespective of the route of administration.

Cysteinyl-leukotrienes are powerful constrictors of human airways in vitro[11,12] through direct interaction with $CysLT_1$ receptors on airway smooth muscle[13], and with a potency at least 1000-fold greater than histamine. In vivo they cause bronchoconstriction both in healthy individuals and in patients with asthma[14] and these responses are inhibited by cys-LT receptor antagonists[15,16]. Interestingly, while the response to inhaled LTC_4 and LTD_4 is exaggerated in asthmatic individuals[14], the differences between normal individuals and patients with bronchial asthma are not as marked as the differences observed with histamine and methacholine. The reasons for this difference between stimuli is at present unclear.

LEUKOTRIENES IN INDUCED AIRWAY CONSTRICTION

Early studies with 5-LO inhibitors and LT receptor antagonists attempted to unravel the role of leukotrienes in various models of asthma, long before such compounds were investigated in phase II trials and even before a clinical application of these drugs was defined. In addition to the extensive literature on allergen provocation, which is covered in another section of these proceedings, other models of induced bronchoconstriction in asthmatics were studied and form the background for this short summary.

Exercise challenge

Cold air and exercise challenge as well as isocapnic hyperventilation studies were among the first models to demonstrate the involvement of LTs in physiological responses in patients with asthma, and to implicate eicosanoids in the pathophysiology of these responses in children[17] and in adults[18–20]. Five-lipoxygenase inhibitors, such as zileuton and ABT-761[21–23], and *CysLT₁* (LTD$_4$) receptor antagonists such as MK-571, LY-171883, zafirlukast, cinalukast, and pobilukast were all shown to inhibit airway constriction in this model[24–30] with a magnitude of effect ranging around 50%, thereby exposing the role of additional mediators in the response to exercise challenge[31]. Along with a considerable individual variability in the protective effect of all LT modifiers studied, there is a marked variability in the duration of protection, depending on the drug used[32,33].

An increase in urinary LTE$_4$ has been demonstrated in children[34], but not in adults, after exercise challenge[35]. In two recent studies, however, a 5-LO inhibitor was shown to significantly suppress urinary LTE$_4$, reflecting the overall decrease in LT production, and both of these independent studies taken together demonstrated an exercise-induced increase in urinary LTE$_4$[22,23].

Aspirin challenge

Aspirin insensitivity is common in adult asthmatic patients (aspirin-induced asthma, AIA) and the pathophysiology and theoretical background of this syndrome will be discussed in detail in another chapter. There is no question that LTs play a major role in this syndrome[36] and that patients with AIA in particular are expected to benefit from treatment with anti-LTs. Clinical trials with 5-LO inhibitors such as zileuton and various LT receptor antagonists such as ONO-1078 (pranlukast) demonstrated significant effects on aspirin-induced bronchoconstriction which in magnitude exceeds the effects seen against allergen and exercise challenge[37–39]. Furthermore, in patients with aspirin intolerance, LT receptor antagonists have a significant effect on baseline lung function, indicating a particular role of abnormal LT production for the clinical presentation of this syndrome[40]. The causal relationship of the beneficial effects of LT modifiers for aspirin intolerance is additionally demonstrated through the findings that these patients exhibit elevated levels of urinary LTE$_4$, and that the clinical improvement is paralleled by a significant overall reduction of LT production after treatment with 5-LO inhibitors[41] as assessed by a decreased excretion of the stable metabolite.

Adenosine challenge

Adenosine has little or no effect on the airway calibre of normal individuals in vivo, but leads to a concentration-related bronchoconstriction in patients with allergic and non-allergic asthma[42]. Similarly, isolated human airways from asthmatics contract in response to adenosine, and this contraction has been shown to be mediated indirectly through the liberation of histamine and LTs[43]. Recently, the first clinical study was undertaken to assess the effect of a 5-LO inhibitor (ABT-761) on adenosine-induced bronchoconstriction in asthmatic patients. In this study the 5-LO inhibitor did not affect the maximal fall in FEV$_1$ after adenosine challenge but inhibited significantly the overall bronchoconstriction. Adenosine caused a 39% increase in urinary LTE$_4$ which was significantly reduced by ABT-761[22].

PAF and SO₂ challenge

Few studies have addressed the role of LTs in other experimental human challenge models of asthma. Two studies have assessed the effect of LT modifiers on platelet activating factor (PAF)-induced bronchoconstriction in humans[44,45] and on changes in airway calibre induced by the environmental pollutant, SO_2[46]. Although LT receptor antagonists inhibited the airway response under these experimental conditions, the significance of the findings is at present unclear since it has so far not been demonstrated that PAF or SO_2 increase LT levels in BAL fluid or that these stimuli increase urinary LTE_4 secretion in man.

CONCLUSIONS

Specific and potent LT receptor antagonists and LT synthesis inhibitors have been shown in clinical trials to be effective against a range of exogenous stimuli which trigger bronchoconstriction in susceptible individuals. Of clinical importance is the protective effect of this class of drugs against allergen challenges, aspirin and exercise. While patients with aspirin idiosyncrasy undoubtedly benefit from LT modifiers, the role for the treatment of exercise-induced bronchoconstriction is more complex, since more than one class of mediators is involved. Since bronchoconstrictor LTs appear to be synthesized in close proximity to human airway smooth muscle, LT modifiers have an additional benefit through their ability to protect against this endogenous contractile stimulus, and this appears particularly relevant in patients with aspirin intolerance.

Whether the observed individual variability in patients in response to LT intervention is due to the existence of certain subgroups of asthmatics where, compared to other mediators, LTs play a more prominent role for the pathophysiology of the disease, or whether genetic variability may determine the individual outcome[47], is at present uncertain. The recent cloning of the LTB_4 receptor[48] may lead to the identification of other classes of LT receptors and, possibly, the recognition of receptor heterogeneity that may help explain the wide variability in clinical responses to LT intervention in patients with asthma.

References

1. Ellis JL, Undem BJ. Role of cysteinyl-leukotrienes and histamine in mediating intrinsic tone in isolated human bronchi. Am J Resp Crit Care Med. 1994; 149: 118–21.
2. Watson N, Magnussen H, Rabe KF. Inherent tone of human bronchus: role of eicosanoids and the bronchial epithelium. Br J Pharmacol. 1997; 121: 1099–104.
3. Peters SP, MacGlashan DW Jr, Schulman ES, et al. Arachidonic acid metabolism in purified human lung mast cells. J Immunol. 1984; 132: 1972–9.
4. Liu MC, Dubé LM, Lancaster J and the zileuton study group. Acute and chronic effects of a 5-lipoxygenase inhibitor in asthma: A 6-month randomized multicenter trial. J Allergy Clin Immunol. 1996; 98: 859–71.
5. Cloud ML, Enas GC, Kemp J, et al. A specific LTD_4/LTE_4-receptor antagonist improves pulmonary function in patients with mild, chronic asthma. Am Rev Resp Dis. 1989; 140: 1336–9.

6. Gaddy JN, Margolskee DJ, Bush RK, Williams VC, Busse WW. Bronchodilation with a potent and selective leukotriene D_4 (LTD_4) receptor antagonist (MK-571) in patients with asthma. Am Rev Resp Dis. 1992; 146: 358–63.

7. Hui KP, Barnes NC. Lung function improvement in asthma with a cysteinyl-leukotriene receptor antagonist. Lancet. 1991; 337: 1062–3.

8. Impens N, Reiss TF, Teahan JA, et al. Acute bronchodilation with an intravenously administered leukotriene D_4 antagonist MK 679. Am Rev Resp Dis. 1993; 147: 1442–6.

9. Lammers JW, Van Daele P, Van Den Elshout FM, et al. Bronchodilator properties of an inhaled leukotriene D_4 antagonist (Verlukast-MK-0679) in asthmatic patients. Pulm Pharmacol. 1992; 5: 121–5.

10. Lockey RF, Lavins BJ, Snader L. Effects of 13 weeks of treatment with ICI 204,219 (Accolate™) in patients with mild to moderate asthma. J. Allergy Clin Immunol. 1995; 95: 350.

11. Dahlén SE, Hedqvist P, Hammaström S, Samuelsson B. Leukotrienes are potent constrictors of human bronchi. Nature. 1980; 228: 484–6.

12. Jones TR, Davis C, Daniel EE. Pharmacological study of the contractile activity of leukotriene C_4 and D_4 on isolated human airway smooth muscle. Can J Physiol Pharmacol. 1982; 60: 638–43.

13. Gorenne I, Norel X, Brink C. Cysteinyl leukotriene receptors in the human lung: What's new? TiPS, 1996; 17: 342–5.

14. Davidson AE, Lee TH, Scanlon PD, Solway J, McFadden ER. Bronchoconstrictor effects of LTE_4 in normal and asthmatic subjects. Am Rev Resp Dis. 1987; 135: 333–7.

15. Shida T, Yui Y. Effect of a selective LT antagonist, ONO-1078, on bronchoconstriction induced by leukotriene D_4 in healthy volunteers. Rinsho Iyaku. 1993; 9 (Suppl. 1): 209–16.

16. Smith LJ, Glass M, Minkwitz MC. Inhibition of leukotriene D_4 induced bronchoconstriction in subjects with asthma: A concentration effect study of ICI 204,219. Clin Pharmacol Ther. 1993; 54: 430–6.

17. Iikura Y, Nagakura T, Walsh GM, et al. Role of chemical mediators after antigen and exercise challenge in children with asthma. J Allergy Clin Immunol. 1988; 81: 1050–5.

18. Broide DH, Eisman S, Ramsdell JW, Ferguson P, Schwartz LB, Wasserman SI. Airway levels of mast cell-derived mediators in exercise-induced asthma. Am Rev Resp Dis. 1990; 141: 563–8.

19. Finnerty JP, Wood-Baker R, Thomson H, Holgate ST. Role of leukotrienes in exercise-induced asthma. Am Rev Resp Dis. 1992; 145: 746–9.

20. Pliss LB, Ingenito EP, Ingram RH, Pichurko B. Assessment of bronchoalveolar cell and mediator response to isocapnic hyperpnea in asthma. Am Rev Resp Dis. 1990; 142: 73–8.

21. Israel E, Dermarkarian R, Rosenberg M, et al. The effects of a 5-lipoxygenase inhibitor on asthma induced by cold, dry air. N Engl J Med. 1990; 323: 1740–4.

22. Van Schoor J, Joos GF, Kips JC, Drajesk JF, Carpentier PJ, Pauwels RA. The effect of ABT-761, a novel 5-lipoxygenase inhibitor, on exercise- and adenosine-induced bronchoconstriction in asthmatic subjects. Am J Resp Crit Care Med. 1997; 155: 875–80.

23. Rabe KF, Lehnigk B, Dent G, Herst PJ, Carpentier PJ, Magnussen H. Exercise-induced bronchoconstriction and urinary LTE_4 levels in patients with bronchial asthma: Effect of ABT-761, a 5-lipoxygenase inhibitor. Eur Resp J. 1995; 8 (Suppl. 19): 473s.

24. Boulet LP, Bai TR, Miller CJ, et al. Effect of zafirlukast on cold-air-induced bronchoconstriction in patients with asthma. Eur Resp J. 1996; 9 (Suppl. 23): 273S.

25. Hirata K, Kurihara N, Kamimori T, Hikiishi F, Fujimoto S, Takeda T. Exercise-induced asthma and leukotriene receptor antagonism. Rinsho Iyaku. 1993; 9 (Suppl. 1): 225–8.

26. Israel E, Juniper EF, Callaghan JT, et al. Effect of a leukotriene antagonist, LY 171883, on cold air-induced bronchoconstriction in asthmatics. Am Rev Resp Dis. 1989; 140: 1348–53.

27. Israel E, Lavins BJ, Miller CJ, Cohn J. Effect of zafirlukast (20 and 40 mg) on cold-air-induced bronchoconstriction in patients with bronchial asthma. Eur Resp J. 1996; 9 (Suppl. 23): 51S.

28. Makker HK, Lau LC, Thomson HW, Binks SM, Holgate ST. The protective effect of inhaled leukotriene D_4 receptor antagonist ICI 204,219 against exercise-induced asthma. Am Rev Resp Dis. 1993; 147: 1413–18.

29. Manning PJ, Watson RM, Margolskee DJ, Williams VC, Schwartz JJ. Inhibition of exercise-induced bronchoconstriction by MK-571, a potent leukotriene D_4 receptor antagonist. N Engl Med. 1990; 323: 1736–9.

30. Robuschi M, Riva E, Fuccella LM, et al. Prevention of exercise-induced bronchoconstriction by a new leukotriene antagonist (SK&F) 104,353. Am Rev Resp Dis. 1992; 145: 1285–8.

31. Finnerty JP, Holgate ST. Evidence for the role of histamine and prostaglandins as mediators in exercise-induced asthma: The inhibitory effect of terfenadine and flurbiprofen alone and in combination. Eur Resp J. 1990; 3: 540–7.

32. Ädelroth E, Inman MD, Summers E, Pace D, Modi M, O'Byrne PM. Prolonged protection against exercise-induced bronchoconstriction by the leukotriene D_4-receptor antagonist cinalukast. J Allergy Clin Immunol. 1997; 99: 210–15.

33. Richter K, Speckin P, Koschyk S, Jörres RA, Magnussen H. Efficacy and duration of action of zafirlukast on cold-air induced bronchoconstriction in patients with asthma. Eur Resp J. 1997; 10: 419S.

34. Kikawa Y, Miyanomae T, Inoue Y, et al. Urinary leukotriene E_4 after exercise challenge in children with asthma. J Allergy Clin Immunol. 1992; 89: 1111–19.

35. Smith CM, Christie PE, Hawksworth RJ, Thien F, Lee TH. Urinary leukotriene E_4 levels after allergen and exercise challenge in bronchial asthma. Am Rev Resp Dis. 1991; 144: 1411–13.

36. Israel E, Fischer AR, Rosenberg MA, et al. The pivotal role of 5-lipoxygenase products in the reaction of aspirin-sensitive asthmatics to aspirin. Am Rev Resp Dis. 1993; 148: 1447–51.

37. Yamamoto H, Nagata M, Kuramitsu K, et al. Inhibition of analgesic-induced asthma by leukotriene receptor antagonist ONO-1078. Am J Resp Crit Care Med. 1994; 150: 254–7.

38. Nasser SM, Bell GS, Foster S, et al. Effects of the 5-lipoxygenase inhibitor ZD 2138 on aspirin-induced asthma. Thorax. 1994; 49: 749–56.

39. Christie PE, Smith CM, Lee TH. The potent and selective sulfidopeptide leukotriene antagonist, SK&F 104,353, inhibits aspirin-induced asthma. Am Rev Resp Dis. 1991; 144: 957–8.

40. Dahlén B, Margolskee DJ, Zetterström O, Dahlén SE. Effect of the leukotriene receptor antagonist MK-0679 on baseline pulmonary function in aspirin sensitive asthmatic subjects. Thorax. 1993; 48: 1205–10.

41. Kumlin M, Dahlén B, Björck T, Zetterström O, Granström E, Dahlén SE. Urinary excretion of leukotrien E_4 and 11-dehydrothromboxane B_2 in response to bronchial provocation with allergen, aspirin, leukotriene D_4 and histamine in asthmatics. Am Rev Resp Dis. 1992; 146: 96–103.

42. Cushley MJ, Tattersfield AE, Holgate ST. Inhaled adenosine and guanosine on airway resistance in normal and asthmatic subjects. Br J Clin Pharmacol. 1983; 15: 161–5.

43. Björck T, Gustafsson LE, Dahlén SE. Isolated bronchi from asthmatics are hyperresponsive to adenosine, which apparently acts indirectly by liberation of leukotrienes and histamine. Am Rev Resp Dis. 1992; 145: 1087–90.

44. Kidney J, Ridge S, Chung KF, Barnes PJ. Inhibition of PAF-induced bronchoconstriction by the oral leukotriene D_4 receptor antagonist, ICI 204,219. Am Rev Resp Dis. 1993; 147: 215–17.

45. Spencer DA, Evans JM, Green SE, Piper PJ, Costello JF. Participation of the cysteinyl leukotrienes in the acute bronchoconstrictor response to inhaled platelet-activating factor in man. Thorax. 1991; 46: 441–5.

46. Lazarus SC, Lavins BJ, Wong HH, Watts MJ, Minkwitz MC. Effect of Accolate™ (zafirlukast) on sulfur dioxide (SO_2)-induced bronchoconstriction in patients with mild to moderate asthma. Allergy. 1995; 50 (Suppl. 26): 45.

47. In Asano K, Beier D, et al. Naturally occurring mutations in the human 5-lipoxygenase gene promoter that modify transcription factor binding and reporter gene transcription. J Clin Invest. 1997; 99: 1130–7.

48. Yokomizo T, Izumi T, Chang K, Takuwa Y, Shimizu T. A G-protein coupled receptor for leukotriene B_4 that mediates chemotaxis. Nature. 1997; 387: 620–4.

9 Role of leukotrienes in aspirin-induced asthma

A. SZCZEKLIK and M. SANAK

Aspirin-induced asthma (AIA) is a well-defined clinical syndrome that affects about 10% of adult asthmatics and in which aspirin and several other non-steroidal anti-inflammatory drugs (NSAID) precipitate asthmatic reactions[1–4]. Although the onset of symptoms before puberty or after the age of 60 has been well documented, in most patients the first symptoms appear during the third or fourth decade of life. Typically, the patient experiences intense vasomotor rhinitis characterized by intermittent and profuse watery rhinorrhoea. Over a period of months or years, chronic nasal congestion appears and physical examination reveals nasal polyps. Bronchial asthma and intolerance to aspirin develop subsequently. The intolerance presents as a unique picture: within an hour after ingestion of aspirin an acute asthma attack develops, often accompanied by rhinorrhoea, conjunctival irritation and scarlet flushing of the head and neck. Aspirin is a common precipitating factor of life-threatening attacks of asthma[5]; in a recent large survey, 25% of asthmatic patients requiring emergency mechanical ventilation were found to be aspirin intolerant[6].

Nasal polyps are a common finding in AIA. They were diagnosed in 47 (61%) of our 80 asthmatic patients with aspirin-intolerance confirmed by provocation tests. Their appearance was preceded by chronic rhinitis, which on average lasted 4 or 5 years, but in some cases up to 21 years. In about 60% of cases the first diagnosis of both aspirin intolerance and bronchial asthma was made prior to diagnosis of nasal polyps.

The asthma runs a protracted course, despite the avoidance of aspirin and cross-reactive drugs. Blood eosinophil count is elevated, and eosinophils are present in airways. The serum IgG4 level is often raised[7] and half of the patients have autoantibodies against ss-DNA at a titre $\geq$ 1:40 in serum[8–10]. Skin tests with aspirin are always negative. Atopy traits, contrary to early reports[1], are not rare: they are, in fact, more common than in the general population[11]. There is a specific pattern of HLA class II antigens, namely a high frequency of DPB*0301, and a low frequency of DPB*0401[12].

Not only aspirin, but several other NSAIDs precipitate attacks. Their chemical structures differ widely, which makes a chemical cross-reactivity most unlikely. Major offenders include indomethacin, fenamic acids, ibuprofen, fenoprofen, ketoprofen, naproxen, diclofenac, piroxicam, tiaprofenic acid, aminopyrine, noramidopyrine, sulfinopyrazone, phenylbutazone and fenflumizole. Not all of these drugs produce adverse symptoms of the same intensity, and the reaction depends on the anticylcooxygenase potency of the drug, dosage and individual sensitivity. If necessary, patients with AIA can safely take sodium salicylate, salicylamide, choline magnesium trisalicylate, dextropropoxyphene, azapropazone and benzidamine. Most patients also tolerate paracetamol well at doses under 1000 μg[13]. Tartrazine, a yellow azo-dye used for colouring drinks, foods, drugs, and cosmetics, very rarely triggers adverse reactions[14].

Although the clinical history of the patient might raise the suspicion of AIA, the diagnosis can be established with certainty only by aspirin challenge. There are no in vitro tests suitable for routine clinical diagnosis, although a search for them continues. There are three types of provocation tests, depending on the route of aspirin administration: oral, inhaled and nasal. Oral challenge tests are the most commonly performed. In inhalation challenge tests an aerosol of lysine-acetylsalicylic acid is administered. Inhalation challenge is faster than the oral challenge, but symptoms evaluated are restricted only to the bronchopulmonary tract. Nasal tests are mainly used in clinical research.

In the majority of patients aspirin intolerance lasts for the rest of the patient's life. Repeated aspirin challenges are therefore positive although some variability in intensity of symptoms occur. In an occasional patient, however, a positive aspirin challenge might become negative after a period of a few years.

THE CYCLOOXYGENASE THEORY

The cyclooxygenase (COX) theory[15] proposes that precipitation of asthma attacks by aspirin is not based on an antigen–antibody reaction, but stems from the pharmacological action of the drug[16]; namely, the specific inhibition in the respiratory tract of the COX enzyme. The original observations[17,18], that the intolerance to the drug can be predicted on the basis of its in vitro inhibition of COX have been consistently reaffirmed over the ensuing years[19,20].

Evidence in favour of the COX theory can be summarized as follows:

1.   NSAIDs with anti-COX activity invariably precipitate bronchoconstriction in aspirin sensitive patients.
2.   NSAIDs that do not affect COX activity do not provoke bronchospasm.
3.   There is a positive correlation between the potency of the NSAID to inhibit COX in vitro and the potency to induce asthma attacks in sensitive patients.
4.   After aspirin desensitization, cross-desensitization to other NSAIDs, which inhibit COX, also occurs.

The enzyme which appears to be central to the mechanism of aspirin intolerance recently became the subject of wide interest[21] when its isoforms were discovered. We now know that COX exists in at least two isoforms, COX-1 and COX-2, which are encoded by distinct genes. The constitutive isoform, COX-1, is expressed in most tissues and has clear physiological functions, while COX-2 is the inducible isoform, produced in response to proinflammatory stimuli in various cells, including human pulmonary epithelial cells, fibroblasts, alveolar macrophages and blood monocytes. Cytokine induction of cytosolic phospholipase A2 and COX-2 mRNA is suppressed by glucocorticoids in epithelial cells.

Aspirin, indomethacin and piroxicam, which at low doses precipitate asthmatic attacks in sensitive patients, are much more potent inhibitors of COX-1 than COX-2. Salicylate is practically devoid of an effect on COX-1 in intact cells, but has half the potency of aspirin in inhibiting COX-2 in certain cell lines. Nimesulide, a drug known to inhibit COX-2 preferentially, was very well tolerated by AIA patients at a dose of 100 mg, but at a higher dose of 400 mg it induced mild pulmonary obstruction[22]. New selective COX inhibitors, which are some 1000-fold more potent against COX-2 than against COX-1, have been synthesized[21]. In experimental animals they display strong anti-inflammatory activity, with few, if any, side effects on stomach or kidney. The introduction of these drugs into the clinic will provide a new, interesting tool for elucidating the relative importance of the COX isoforms in AIA.

RELEASE OF CYSTEINYL-LEUKOTRIENES AND OTHER MEDIATORS

In AIA inhibition of COX is associated with release of cysteinyl-leukotrienes (cys-LTs). Their biological effects[23,24] are consistent with most symptoms observed in AIA. Furthermore, the eosinophil and the mast cell, two cells that play an essential role in AIA, can produce large quantities of cys-LTs. Some patients with AIA excrete 2–10 times more LTE_4 in urine than do other asthmatics who tolerate aspirin well. However, when baseline urinary LTE_4 levels in 10 AIA patients were compared to those in 31 aspirin-tolerant asthmatics[25] there was a substantial overlap between the groups, and no correlation was found between urinary LTE_4 and histamine PD_{20} or baseline forced expiratory volume in 1 s (FEV_1). There is no doubt that aspirin challenge results in a temporary, though significant, increase in urinary LTE_4 excretion[26–28] (Figure 1). Cys-LTs are also released into the nasal cavity after nasal challenge with aspirin[29–32], and into bronchi after inhalation challenge with lysine-aspirin[33]. This is accompanied by inhibition of TXB_2 and prostaglandin (PGE_2) production, while 15-lipoxygenase (LO) metabolites remain unaltered[31].

Local instillation of aspirin in the nose or bronchi of the sensitive patients followed by nasal washing or bronchoalveolar lavage (BAL) allows one to investigate the tissue response to aspirin and the course of the reaction. Kowalski et al.[33] reported that intranasal challenge with aspirin led to increased vascular permeability and an early influx of eosinophils into nasal secretions of aspirin intolerant patients. This was accompanied by an increase in concentrations of eosinophil cationic protein and tryptase, and development of clinical symptoms, consisting of rhinorrhoea, sneezing and nasal congestion. No changes were detected in nasal washings of the asthmatic patients who tolerated aspirin well. Cysteinyl-LTs were not measured in this study, but their enhanced release has been demonstrated convincingly in previous reports[30–32]. However, studies of the release of histamine and PGD_2 yielded inconsistent results. Some authors[34] reported a marked rise in levels of these two mediators in nasal washings after oral aspirin challenge, while others[32] did not confirm these results. Studies in atopic patients indicate that PGD_2 measurement in nasal secretion might not be a reliable marker for mast cell activation[35].

Segmental bronchial challenge with aspirin has been recently performed in two well matched groups of patients: AIA and asthmatics tolerant of aspirin[36]. At baseline

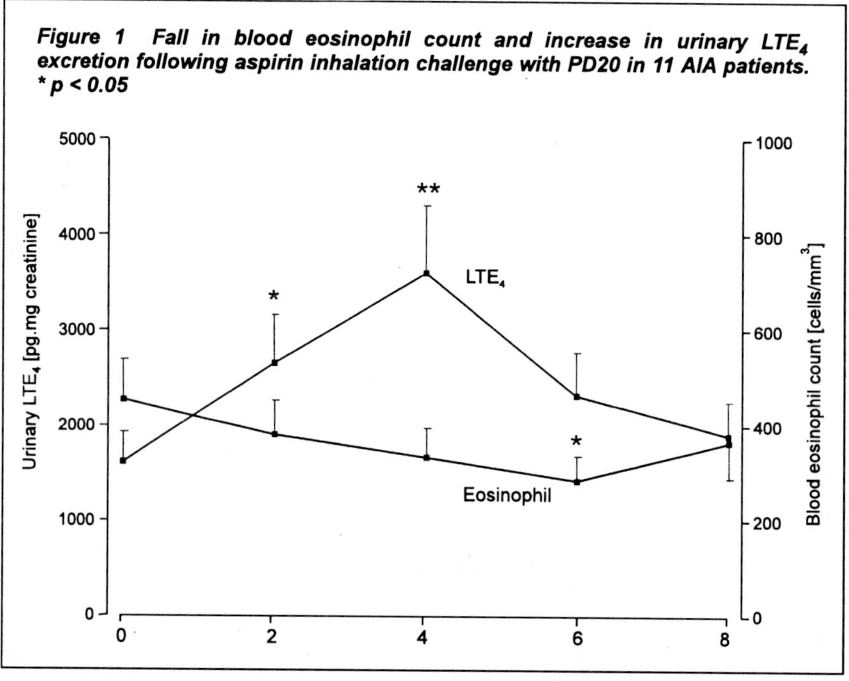

*Figure 1   Fall in blood eosinophil count and increase in urinary LTE$_4$ excretion following aspirin inhalation challenge with PD20 in 11 AIA patients. * p < 0.05*

the two groups did not differ in the BAL fluid concentrations of COX products, cys-LTs, histamine, tryptase, interleukin-5 (IL-5) or eosinophil count. Fifteen minutes after intrabronchial instillation of 10 mg L-lysine aspirin, there was a statistically significant rise in cys-LTs (Figure 2), IL-5 and eosinophil count in the BAL fluid of AIA, but not of aspirin-tolerant patients. Mean histamine concentrations rose in response to aspirin, approaching the level of statistical significance. Aspirin significantly depressed PGE_2 and TXB_2 in both groups, however mean PGD_2, $PGF_{2\alpha}$ and $9\alpha,11\beta$-PGF_2 decreased only in aspirin-tolerant patients. In individual AIA subjects, PGD_2 levels showed variability in response to aspirin, from a marked increase to depression. Interestingly, Warren et al.[37] reported that segmental bronchial challenge with indomethacin led to a rise in PGD_2 and histamine in BAL fluid of three aspirin-sensitive asthmatics, in contrast to three aspirin-tolerant asthmatics. Thus, bronchial aspirin challenge causes a specific eicosanoid response in aspirin-sensitive asthmatics. By removing bronchodilator PGE_2 and leaving unchecked bronchoconstrictor PGD_2 and $PGF_{2\alpha}$, aspirin might further tip the eicosanoid balance towards bronchial obstruction, a balance already disturbed by cys-LT overproduction (Figure 3).

ENZYMES CONTROLLING LEUKOTRIENE AND PROSTANOID BIOSYNTHESIS PATHWAYS

During stimulus-specific cell activation, arachidonic acid released by cytosolic phospholipase A_2 ($cPLA_2$) and translocated to the 5-lipoxygenase activating protein

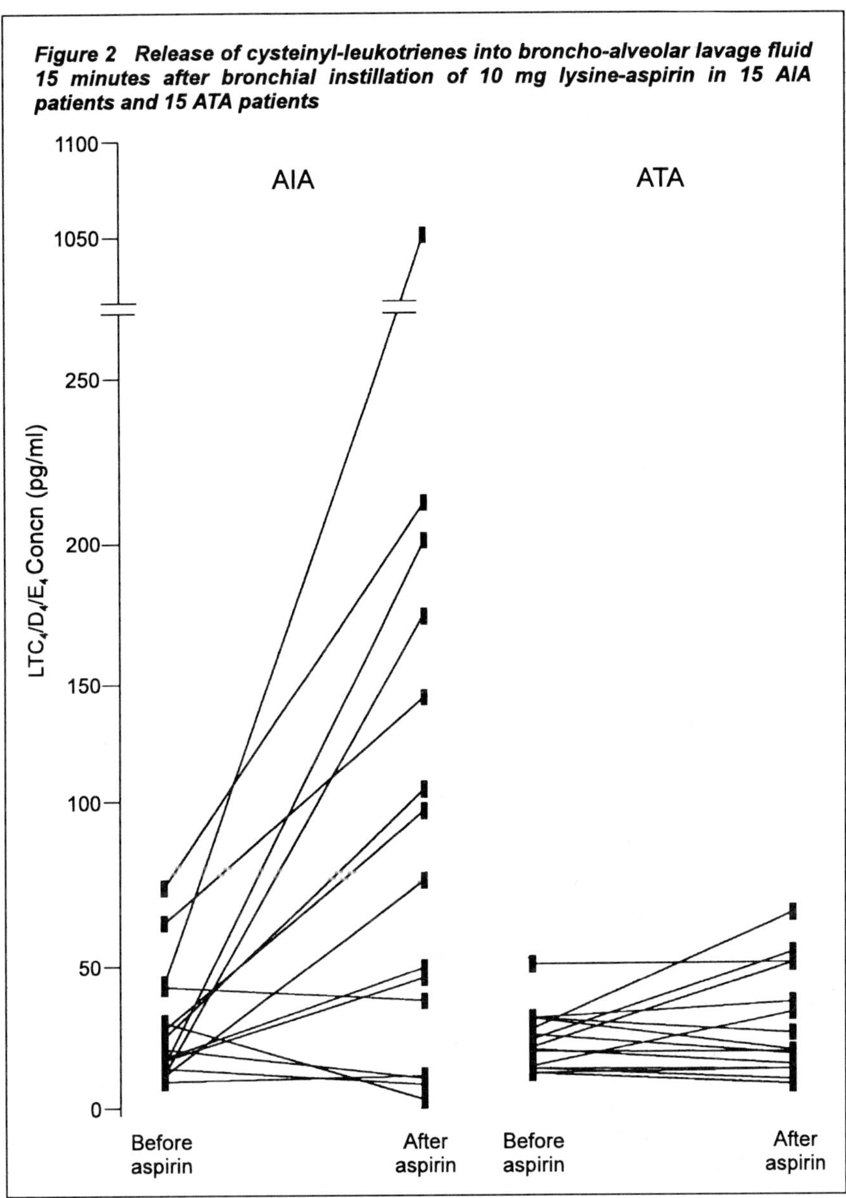

Figure 2 *Release of cysteinyl-leukotrienes into broncho-alveolar lavage fluid 15 minutes after bronchial instillation of 10 mg lysine-aspirin in 15 AIA patients and 15 ATA patients*

(FLAP) is converted in two steps to leukotriene (LT) A$_4$ by 5-lipoxygenase (5-LO). LTA$_4$ is converted to the dihydroxy leukotriene, LTB$_4$ by cells expressing LTA$_4$ hydrolase, and/or to the cysteinyl leukotriene, LTC$_4$, by cells expressing LTC$_4$ synthase, which conjugates LTA$_4$ to reduced glutathione. After carrier-mediated cellular export

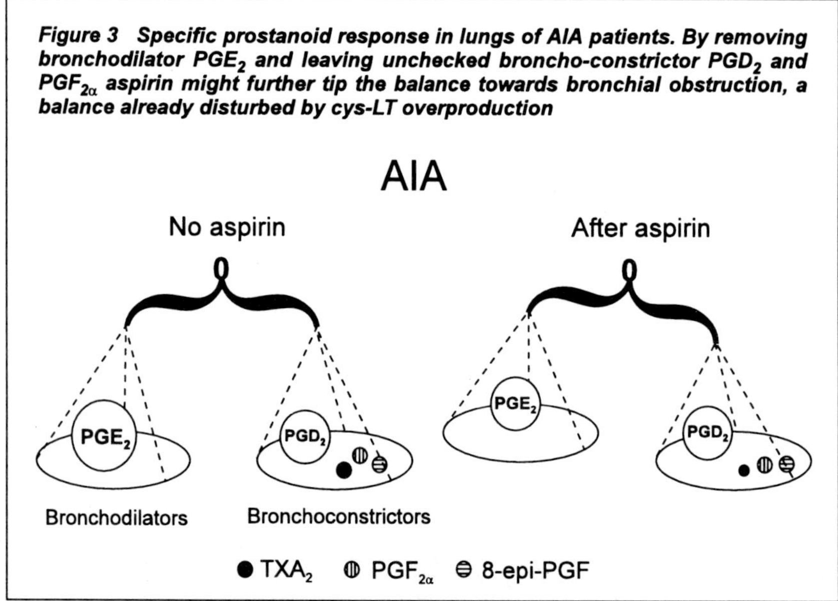

Figure 3   Specific prostanoid response in lungs of AIA patients. By removing bronchodilator PGE$_2$ and leaving unchecked broncho-constrictor PGD$_2$ and PGF$_{2\alpha}$ aspirin might further tip the balance towards bronchial obstruction, a balance already disturbed by cys-LT overproduction

of LTC$_4$, the sequential cleavage of Glu and Gly provides the extracellular, receptor-active metabolites LTD$_4$ and LTE$_4$ respectively.

The 5-LO/LTC$_4$ synthase pathway is limited to cells of bone marrow origin, and the chronic defect subject to exacerbation with aspirin challenge could be the over-expression of some step in the LT synthetic pathway in the infiltrating eosinophils/basophils or resident mast cells/macrophages. Alternatively, or in addition, there could be under-representation of some control function of the prostanoid pathways, which are widely distributed in diverse lineage cell types. In prostanoid biosynthesis, the released arachidonic acid is directly converted by constitutive COX-1 or by induced COX-2 in two steps to the intermediate PGH$_2$, which is common to the terminal prostanoid synthases and thromboxane synthase.

In a recent study[38] we identified and quantified the cells expressing the principal enzymes of the COX and 5-LO pathways in biopsies of bronchial mucosa from patients with AIA, ATA and non-atopic normal individuals. We confirmed the previous report[39] that immunostaining for COX-1, COX-2 and 5-LO in bronchial biopsies from AIA and ATA patients is not different, and extended this finding to FLAP and LTA$_4$ hydrolase and even to a comparison with normal subjects. In contrast, there is a profound over-representation of cells expressing LTC$_4$ synthase, the integral perinuclear membrane enzyme that forms LTC$_4$, the intracellular parent of the released receptor-active cleavage products LTC$_4$ and LTE$_4$, in AIA bronchial biopsies compared to cells expressing the enzyme in biopsies from ATA and normal individuals. This unique difference may provide a basis for the chronic over-production and for the aspirin-induced increase in cys-LT production in AIA, and for the lack of adverse responses to NSAIDs in ATA patients and normal subjects.

The predominant population of LTC_4 synthase cells were eosinophils, only a small proportion being mast cells and macrophages. LTC_4 synthase-positive cell numbers in the bronchial submucosa correlated with basal levels of cys-LTs in BAL fluid, suggesting that higher numbers of LTC_4 synthase-positive cells may explain chronic cys-LT over-production and impaired baseline lung function in AIA patients.

The immunohistochemical differences at baseline between AIA and ATA patient groups were highlighted by a 4-fold increase in eosinophils, a 5-fold increase in LTC_4 synthase cells (predominantly eosinophils) and a 4-fold increase in IL-5+ cells (predominantly mast cells). Since the gene for human LTC_4 synthase resides on the long arm of chromosome 5, distal to the gene cluster which regulates the development and function of the T2 cells, namely IL-4, IL-13, IL-3, IL-5, GM-CSF and IL-9, a polymorphism directed to the regulation of LTC_4 synthase expression could be a predisposing factor for AIA.

ANTI-LEUKOTRIENE DRUGS

Proof of the critical role of cys-LTs in AIA has been provided by the advent of anti-LT drugs. These compounds either inhibit LT synthesis by blocking 5-LO or its activator, 5-LO-activating protein (FLAP), or block specific cys-LT receptors. Premedication with LT synthesis inhibitors or cys-LT-receptor antagonists cause marked attenuation of aspirin-precipitated nasal and bronchial reactions[34,40–42], while histamine antagonists have little effect[43,44]. Bronchodilation has also been observed with anti-LT agents, indicating that cys-LTs have an effect on intrinsic airway tone in AIA.

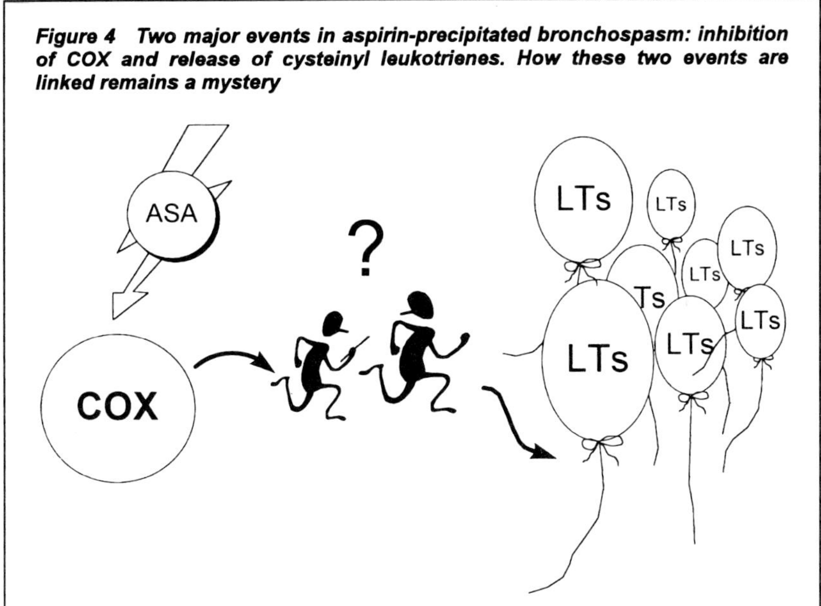

Figure 4   Two major events in aspirin-precipitated bronchospasm: inhibition of COX and release of cysteinyl leukotrienes. How these two events are linked remains a mystery

Anti-LT drugs might soon find a place in the chronic treatment of AIA. In a Swedish–Polish placebo-controlled, crossover study[45] 40 AIA patients received 6 weeks' treatment with the 5-LO inhibitor, zileuton, or placebo. Zileuton produced a significant improvement in airway function, decrease in nasal obstruction, return of the sense of smell, and reduction in airway responsiveness to histamine. A recently concluded, double-blind, placebo-controlled, parallel-group, 4-week study[46] assessed the therapeutic effects of montelukast or placebo once daily at bedtime. Patients on montelukast had significant improvement in parameters of asthma control, including FEV_1 and PEFR.

CONCLUSIONS

There is now good evidence that aspirin-precipitated asthmatic reactions result from inhibition of COX that is accompanied by release of cys-LTs. Eosinophils appear to be the best candidates for the cellular source of cys-LTs, while activation of mast cells is also likely to affect the course of the reaction. The basis of the link between COX-inhibition and LT overproduction remains elusive (Figure 4), though interesting suggestions have been recently advanced. Little is known about the cause of the disease, which is acquired and runs a chronic course, even when NSAIDs are avoided. Search for the predisposing factors, especially of immunological origin, for aberrations in intracellular signal transduction, for polymorphism of genes controlling prostaglandin and leukotriene biosynthesis and for a virus as a possible principle initiating and promoting the disease, might lead to the solution of the enigma presented by this clinical syndrome.

References

1. Samter M, Beers RF. Intolerance to aspirin. Clinical studies and consideration of its pathogenesis. Ann Intern Med. 1968; 68: 975–83.
2. Stevenson DD. Diagnosis, prevention and treatment of adverse reactions to aspirin and nonsteroidal anti-inflammatory drugs. J Allergy Clin Immunol. 1984; 74: 617–22.
3. Szczeklik A. Aspirin-induced asthma. In: Vane JR, Botting RM, editors. Aspirin and other salicylates. London: Chapman and Hall Medical, 1992: 548–75.
4. Szczeklik A. Mechanism of aspirin-induced asthma. Allergy. 1997; 52: 613–19.
5. Picado C, Castillo JA, Montserrat JM, Augusti-Vidal A. Aspirin-intolerance as a precipitating factor of life-threatening attacks of asthma requiring mechanical ventilation. Eur Resp J. 1989; 2: 127–9.
6. Marquette CH, Saulnier F, Leroy O, et al. Long-term prognosis for near-fatal asthma. A 6-year follow-up study of 145 asthmatic patients who underwent mechanical ventilation for near-fatal attack of asthma. Am Rev Resp Dis. 1992; 146: 76–81.
7. Szczeklik A, Schmitz-Schumann M, Niżankowska E, Milewski M, Roehlig F, Virchow C. Altered distribution of IgG subclasses in aspirin-induced asthma: high IgG4, low IgG1. Clin Exp Allergy. 1992; 22: 283–7.
8. Szczeklik A, Niżankowska E, Serafin A, Dyczek A, Duplaga M, Musial J. Autoimmune phenomena in bronchial asthma with special reference to aspirin intolerance. Am J Resp Crit Care Med. 1995; 152: 1753–6.
9. Lasalle P, Delneste Y, Gosset P, Grass-Masse H, Wallaert B, Tonnel AB. T and B cell immune response to a 55-kDa endothelial cell-derived antigen in severe asthma. Eur J Immunol. 1993; 23: 796–803.

10. Szczeklik A, Musial J, Pulka G. Autoimmune vasculitis and aortic stenosis in aspirin-induced asthma. Allergy. 1997; 52: 352–4.

11. Bochenek G. Niżankowska E, Szczeklik A. Atopy trait in hypersensitivity to nonsteroidal anti-inflammatory drugs. Allergy. 1996; 51: 16–23.

12. Dekker JW, Niżankowska E, Schmitz-Schumann M, et al. Aspirin-induced asthma and HLA-DRB1 and HLA-DPB1 genotypes. Clin Exp Allergy. 1997; 27: 574–7.

13. Settipane RA, Schrank PJ, Simon RA, Mathison DA, Christiansen SC, Stevenson DD. Prevalence of cross-sensitivity with acetaminophen in aspirin-sensitive asthmatic subjects. J Allergy Clin Immunol. 1995; 96: 480–5.

14. Virchow Ch, Szczeklik A, Bianco S, et al. Intolerance to tartrazine in aspirin-induced asthma: results of a multicenter study. Respiration. 1988; 53: 20–3.

15. Szczeklik A. The cyclooxygenase theory of aspirin-induced asthma. Eur Resp J. 1990; 3: 588–93.

16. Vane JR. Inhibition of prostaglandin synthesis as a mechanism of action for aspirin-like drugs. Nature. 1971; 231: 232–4.

17. Szczeklik A, Gryglewski RJ, Czerniawska-Mysik G. Clinical patterns of hypersensitivity to nonsteroidal antiinflammatory drugs and their pathogenesis. J Allergy Clin Immunol. 1977; 60: 276–84.

18. Szczeklik A, Gryglewski RJ, Czerniawska-Mysik G. Relationship of inhibition of prostaglandin biosynthesis by analgesics to asthma attacks in aspirin-sensitive patients. BMJ. 1975; 1: 67–9.

19. Stevenson DD, Lewis RA. Proposed mechanisms of aspirin sensitivity reactions. J Allergy Clin Immunol. 1987; 80: 788–90.

20. Lee TH. Mechanism of aspirin sensitivity. Am Rev Resp Dis. 1992; 145: 34–6.

21. Bazan N, Botting J, Vane JR. New targets in inflammation. Inhibitors of COX-2 or adhesion molecules. Dordrecht: Kluwer and William Harvey Press, 1996.

22. Bianco S, Robuschi M, Petrigni G, et al. Efficacy and tolerability of nimesulide in asthmatic patients intolerant to aspirin. Drugs. 1993; 46 (suppl. 1): 115–20.

23. Busse WW. The role of leukotrienes in asthma and allergic rhinitis. Clin Exp Allergy. 1996; 26: 868–79.

24. Sampson AP. The leukotrienes: Mediators of chronic inflammation in asthma. Clin Exp Allergy. 1996; 26: 995–1004.

25. Smith CM, Hawksworth RJ, Thien FC, Christie PE, Lee TH. Urinary leukotriene E4 in bronchial asthma. Eur Resp J. 1992; 5: 693–9.

26. Christie PE, Tagari P, Ford-Hutchinson AW, Charlesson S, Chee P, Arm JP, Lee TH. Urinary leukotriene E_4 concentrations increase after aspirin challenge in aspirin-sensitive asthmatic subjects. Am Rev Resp Dis. 1991, 143: 1025–9.

27. Kumlin M, Dahlén B, Bjorck T, Zetterstrom O, Granstrom E, Dahlén SE. Urinary excretion of leukotriene E_4 and 11-dehydro-thromboxane B_2 in response to provocations with allergen, aspirin, leukotriene D_4 and histamine in asthmatics. Am Rev Resp Dis. 1992; 146: 96–103.

28. Sladek K, Szczeklik A. Cysteinyl leukotrienes overproduction and mast cell activation in aspirin-provoked bronchospasm in asthma. Eur Resp J. 1993; 6: 391–9.

29. Ortolani C, Mirone C, Fontana A, et al. Study of mediators of anaphylaxis in nasal wash fluids after aspirin and sodium metabisulfite nasal provocation in intolerant rhinitic patients. Ann Allergy. 1987; 59: 106–12.

30. Ferreri NR, Howland WC, Stevenson DD, Spiegelberg HL. Release of leukotrienes, prostaglandins and histamine into nasal secretions of aspirin-sensitive asthmatic during reaction to aspirin. Am Rev Resp Dis. 1988; 137: 847–54.

31. Picado C, Ramis I, Rosello J, et al. Release of peptido-leukotrienes into nasal secretions after local instillation of aspirin in aspirin-sensitive asthmatic patients. Am Rev Resp Dis. 1992; 145: 65–9.

32. Kowalski ML, Sliwinska-Kowalska M, et al. Nasal secretions in response to acetylsalicylic acid. J Allergy Clin Immunol. 1993; 91: 580–98.

33. Kowalski ML, Grzegorczyk J, Wojciechowska B, Poniatowska M. Intranasal challenge with aspirin induces cell influx and activation of eosinophils and mast cells in nasal secretions of ASA-sensitive patients. Clin Exp Allergy. 1996; 26: 807–14.

34. Fischer AR, Rosenberg MA, Lilly CM, et al. Direct evidence for a role of the mast cell in the nasal response to aspirin in aspirin-sensitive asthma. J Allergy Clin Immunol. 1994; 94: 1046–56.
35. Wong D-Y, Smitz J, Clement P. Prostaglandin D2 measurement in nasal secretions is not a reliable marker for mast cell activation in atopic patients. Clin Exp Allergy. 1995; 25: 1228–34.
36. Szczeklik A, Sladek K, Dworski R, et al. Bronchial aspirin challenge causes specific eicosanoid response in aspirin sensitive asthmatics. Am J Resp Crit Care Med. 1996; 154: 1608–14.
37. Warren MS, Sloan SJ, Westcott JY, Hamilos D, Wenzel SE. LTE$_4$ increases in bronchoalveolar lavage fluid (BALF) of aspirin-intolerant asthmatics (AIA) after instillation of indomethacin. J Allergy Clin Immunol. 1995; 95: 170.
38. Sampson AP, Coburn AS, Sladek K, et al. Profound overexpression of leukotriene C$_4$ synthase in aspirin-intolerant asthmatic bronchial biopsies. Int Arch Allergy Immunol. 1977; 113: 355–7.
39. Nasser SMS, Pfister R, Christie PE, et al. Inflammatory cell populations in bronchial biopsies from aspirin-sensitive asthmatic subjects. Am J Resp Crit Care Med. 1996; 153: 90–6.
40. Christie PE, Smith CM, Lee TH. The potent and selective sulfidopeptide leukotriene antagonist, SK&F 104353, inhibits aspirin-induced asthma. Am Rev Resp Dis. 1991; 144: 957–8.
41. Dahlén B, Margolskee DJ, Zetterstrom O, Dahlén S-E. Effect of the leukotriene receptor antagonist MK-0679 on baseline pulmonary function in aspirin sensitive asthmatic subjects. Thorax. 1993; 48: 1205–10.
42. Yamamoto H, Nagata M, Kuramitsu K, et al. Inhibition of analgesic-induced asthma by leukotriene receptor antagonist ONO-1078. Am J Resp Crit Care Med. 1994; 150: 254–7.
43. Szczeklik A, Serwonska M. Inhibition of idiosyncratic reactions to aspirin in asthmatic patients by clemastine. Thorax. 1979; 34: 654–7.
44. Philips GD, Foord R, Holgate ST. Inhaled lysine-aspirin as a bronchoprovocation procedure in aspirin-sensitive asthma: Its repeatability absence of a late-phase reaction and the role of histamine. J Allergy Clin Immunol. 1989; 84: 232–41.
45. Dahlén S-E, Niżankowska E, Dahlén B, et al. The Swedish-Polish treatment study with the 5-lipoxygenase inhibitor Zileuton in aspirin-intolerant asthmatics. Am J Resp Crit Care Med. 1995; 151: A376.
46. Kuna P, Malmström K, Dahlén S-E, et al. Montelukast (MK-0476), a cys-LT1 receptor antagonist, improves asthma control in aspirin-intolerant asthmatic patients. Am J Resp Crit Care Med. 1997; 155: A975.

10 How to use anti-leukotrienes in the treatment of asthma

J. C. KIPS and R. A. PAUWELS

Asthma is currently defined as a chronic inflammatory disease of the airways. The goals of proper asthma therapy, as put forward in recent guidelines, are not only to prevent symptoms and exacerbations, but also to allow for normal activity levels and maintain pulmonary function within near normal limits[1]. In order to achieve these goals, a stepwise therapeutic approach has been adopted. This is based on obvious avoidance measures, in combination with pharmacological intervention. Medication used for asthma treatment is broadly categorized into two classes: long-term medication, used to achieve and maintain control of the disease, and immediate relief medication, used to treat acute symptoms and exacerbations.

LEUKOTRIENES IN ASTHMA

Ideally, control medication should achieve its effect by interfering with key chemical mediators involved in the pathophysiology of the disease. Sulfidopeptide leukotrienes (LT) appear to fulfil particularly well the criteria as a potential target in the treatment of asthma (Table 1, Figure 1). First, they are present in increased amounts in asthmatic airways[2]; second, they have been shown to be not only potent bronchoconstrictor agonists, but also to have important pro-inflammatory effects [3–5]. In addition, their potential role in the pathogenesis of structural airway changes observed in chronic asthma is increasingly being recognized [6, 7]. Third, specific LT receptor antagonists have proven beneficial effects in asthmatic subjects: even administration of a single dose causes bronchodilatation in mild to moderate asthma, indicating that LTs contribute to baseline airway calibre in these patients[8–10]. Anti-LTs also protect against a variety of bronchoconstrictor stimuli, including allergens[11–15].

The anti-inflammatory potential of anti-LTs in asthma has been confirmed in a number of studies. Zileuton, a 5-lipoxygenase (5-LO) inhibitor, inhibits allergen-induced eosinophil influx into the airways and attenuates the fall in FEV_1, together with the increase in eosinophil numbers and LT levels in bronchoalveolar lavage (BAL) fluid observed during nocturnal asthma[16,17]. Calhoun et al. similarly reported that pretreatment with zafirlukast inhibits the BAL eosinophilia induced by endobronchial allergen challenge[18]. Chronic treatment with montelukast, another potent *CysLT₁* receptor antagonist, decreases both circulating and sputum eosinophil counts in patients with mild uncontrolled asthma[19]. Based on these observations, it seems reasonable to anticipate that anti-LTs could constitute a useful development in control medication.

89

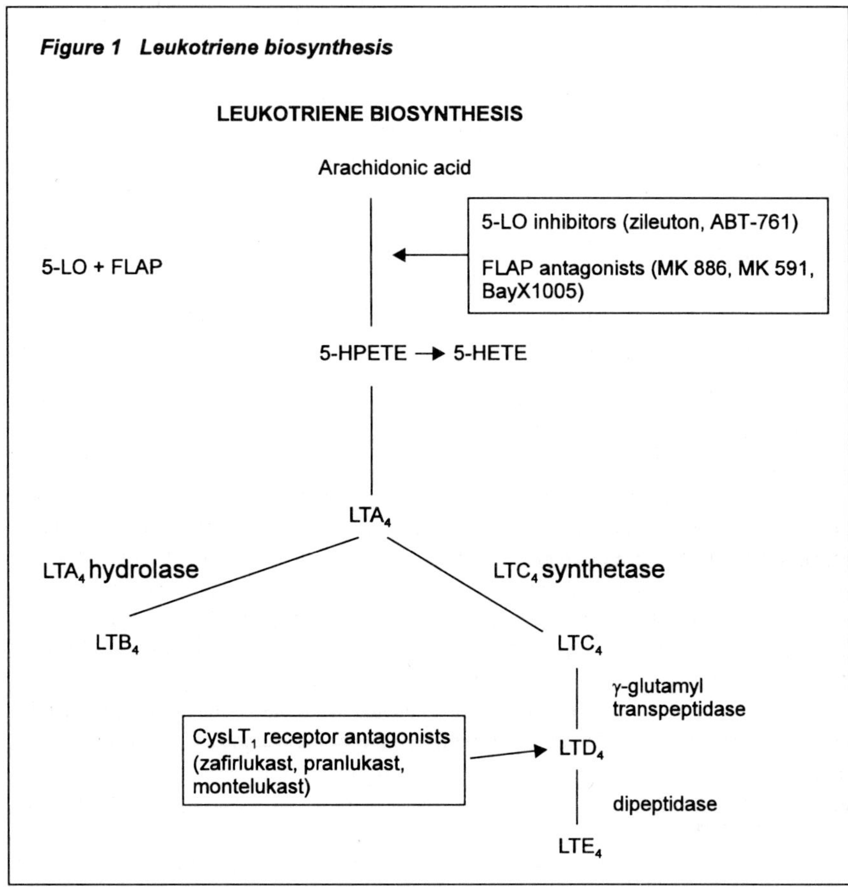

Table 1 Biological properties of leukotrienes, relevant to asthma

Potent bronchoconstrictor (100 – 1000 x histamine or methacholine)
Increase in microvascular permeability
Vasodilatation
Increase in mucus production
Sensitization to other bronchoconstrictor agonists
Recruitment of granulocytes into the airways
Facilitation of airway smooth muscle proliferation

ANTI-LEUKOTRIENES AS CONTROL MEDICATION IN ASTHMA

The effectiveness of anti-LTs as a control medication has been addressed in a number of clinical studies. Initial studies were conducted in patients with mild to moderate asthma, treated with short-acting β_2-agonists only. In this patient population, 6 months' treatment with the 5-LO inhibitor zileuton at a dose of 1.6 or 2.4 g/day was compared to placebo. The highest dose of zileuton resulted in a significant increase in baseline FEV_1 (15% versus 7% in the placebo group), improvement in peak flow recordings and a decrease in symptoms and in β_2-agonist use. The treatment was well tolerated; adverse events were similar in the three groups[20]. Zafirlukast, pranlukast and montelukast are selective *CysLT*$_1$ receptor antagonists that are currently approved for use in a number of countries. Treatment with pranlukast for 12 weeks produced a small, non-dose dependent improvement in peak flow and symptom score over placebo[21]. Treatment with zafirlukast 20 mg bid for 6 or 13 weeks also produced clinical improvement, and a small but significant increase in FEV_1. Again the treatment was well tolerated[22–24]. Compared with placebo, montelukast, 10 mg once daily over 3 months, increased baseline FEV_1 significantly (13.5 vs. 4%), improved quality of life and increased the number of asthma-free days. The need for oral corticosteroid rescue and the number of asthma exacerbations were reduced. The treatment was generally well tolerated[25].

Overall, these studies illustrate that chronic treatment with anti-LTs offers a significant clinical benefit, without apparent side effects in patients with mild to moderate asthma.

An obvious question is how this compares to the effect of other control medications such as chromones or inhaled corticosteroids in this type of patient. These comparative studies are currently ongoing. Preliminary data indicate that 12 weeks' treatment with pranlukast (up to 450 mg bid) induces a comparable clinical improvement to nedocromil (3.5 mg qid). In addition, pranlukast slightly but significantly improved FEV_1 compared with placebo[26]. In another comparative study, zafirlukast 20 mg bid had similar efficacy to cromolyn (2 puffs qid)[27].

Comparative data with inhaled corticosteroids are equally sparse. Pranlukast 450 mg bid, given for 12 weeks, or beclomethasone diproprionate (BDP) 84 μg qid were recently reported to have similar effects on peak flow, symptom score and β_2-agonist use in a group of 417 patients. Notably, only BDP produced a significant improvement in FEV_1[28].

These very limited data would seem to suggest that anti-LTs have similar efficacy to chromones in the treatment of mild to moderate asthma. However, additional comparative data are needed before any firm conclusion can be made. This applies even more so for the comparison with inhaled steroids.

Important issues that need to be addressed in these comparative studies include not only the assessment of benefit over side effect ratio, but also a pharmaco-economic evaluation and the issue of patient compliance. It has to be remembered that the currently developed anti-LTs are all orally formulated, most of them to be taken twice daily although only once daily in the case of montelukast. This might influence patient compliance favourably, in comparison to inhaled formulations. Additional questions that need to be resolved for the exact value of anti-LTs, especially in moderate to severe asthma, is whether adding these compounds has a beneficial effect in patients already treated with inhaled steroids or, conversely, whether this would allow a reduction in the dose of inhaled steroids. Again, only a limited amount of information is currently available in this regard. Recently, a steroid withdrawal study, comparing the effect of pranlukast to placebo over a 6-week period in 83 moderate to severe asthmatics, was published. All patients were on inhaled steroids at a daily dose of at least 1500 µg beclomethasone. Adding pranlukast, as opposed to placebo, allowed the dose of inhaled steroids to be halved, without causing deterioration in symptom score, lung function, serum ECP or exhaled NO levels[29]. Other studies have failed to confirm that adding zafirlukast allows reduction in the dose of inhaled steroids in patients with moderate asthma[30,31]. However, as steroid withdrawal studies are fraught with methodological difficulties, the interpretation of these data is not always straightforward.

Limited data from a preliminary add-on study indicate that adding zileuton, 600 mg qid, to inhaled beclomethasone (200 µg bid) over a 3-month period is as effective for asthma control as BDP 400 µg bid alone[32].

Finally, anti-LTs could be particularly beneficial in specific subgroups of asthma patients. Various lines of evidence indicate that LTs play a predominant role in the pathophysiology of aspirin-sensitive asthma [33–36]. In line with this observation, it was recently reported that 4-weeks' treatment with montelukast, 10 mg daily, improves asthma control in aspirin-sensitive asthmatic patients, incompletely controlled with corticosteroids[37]. It seems plausible that asthma is a heterogeneous disease and that the relative pathophysiological importance of a given inflammatory mediator varies substantially between individual patients. Early studies evaluating the effect of anti-LTs on baseline airway calibre or examining their protective effect against a variety of challenges such as exercise revealed quite a large inter-individual variability in the response observed. This suggests that some asthmatic subjects are indeed more 'leukotriene-driven' than others. However, from these studies no clear pattern has emerged that would enable one to predict the individual response to anti-LTs. As clinical experience with this new group of compounds increases it will be interesting to observe whether other characteristic features will become recognizable, allowing one to identify those asthmatic subjects whose symptoms depend upon markedly raised LT levels.

CONCLUSIONS

Current clinical experience with anti-LTs underlines the potential of this new class of compounds as a control medication in the treatment of asthma. However, the precise indications for the use of anti-LTs within the overall group of available treatment regimens remain to be fully established. Recently published British Thoracic Society guidelines consider the currently available information insufficient for the proper clinical positioning of these compounds at present[38]. The updated 1997 American NIH guidelines on the other hand have positioned anti-LTs as a possible alternative for the treatment of mild, persistent asthma in patients over 12 years of age. However, low doses in inhaled steroids or chromones are still considered the preferred treatment in this patient group[39].

Growing clinical experience with these compounds will undoubtedly allow further establishment of their exact value for the treatment of asthma.

References

1. GINA report. International Consensus report on diagnosis and management of asthma. US Dept Health and Human Services, 1992.

2. Lam S, Chan H, Leriche JC, Chan-Yeung M, Salari H. Release of leukotrienes in patients with bronchial asthma. J Allergy Clin Immunol. 1988; 81: 711–17.

3. Adelroth E, Morris MM, Hargreave FE, O'Byrne P. Airway responsiveness to leukotrienes C_4 and D_4 and to methacholine in patients with asthma and normal controls. N Engl J Med. 1986; 315: 480–4.

4. Drazen JM, Austen KF. Leukotrienes and airway responses. Am Rev Resp Dis. 1987; 136: 985–98.

5. Laitinen LA, Laitinen A, Haahtela T, Vilkka V, Spur BW, Lee TH. Leukotriene E_4 and granulocytic infiltration into asthmatic airways. Lancet. 1993; 341: 989–90.

6. Hay DWP, Torphy TJ, Undem BJ. Cysteinyl leukotrienes in asthma: Old mediators up to new tricks. TiPS. 1995; 16: 304–09.

7. Cohen P, Noveral JP, Bhala A, Nunn SE, Herrick DJ, Grunstein MM. Leukotriene D_4 facilitates airway smooth muscle cell proliferation via modulation of the IGF axis. Am J Physiol. 1995; 269: L151–7.

8. Gaddy JN, Margolskee DJ, Bush RK, Williams VC, Busse WW. Bronchodilation with a potent and selective leukotriene D_4 (LTD_4) receptor antagonist (MK-571) in patients with asthma. Am Rev Resp Dis. 1992; 146: 358–63.

9. Hui KP, Barnes NC. Lung function improvement in asthma with a cysteinyl-leukotriene receptor antagonist. Lancet. 1991; 337: 1062–3.

10. Reiss TF, Sorkness CA, Stricker W, et al. Effects of montelukast (MK-0476), a potent cysteinyl leukotriene receptor antagonist, on bronchodilation in asthmatic subjects treated with and without inhaled corticosteroids. Thorax. 1997; 52: 45–8.

11. Israel E, Juniper EF, Callaghan JT, et al. Effect of a leukotriene antagonist, LY 171883 on cold air-induced bronchoconstriction in asthmatics. Am Rev Resp Dis. 1989; 140: 1348–53.

12. Manning PJ, Watson RM, Margolskee DJ, Williams VC, Schwartz JI, O'Byrne PM. Inhibition of exercise-induced bronchoconstriction by MK-571, a potent leukotriene D_4-receptor antagonist. N Engl J Med 1990; 323: 1736–9.

13. Finnerty JP, Wood-Baker R, Thomson H, Holgate ST. Role of leukotrienes in exercise-induced asthma. Am Rev Resp Dis. 1992; 145: 746–9.

14. Taylor IK, O'Shaughnessy KM, Fuller RW, Dollery CT. Effect of cysteinyl-leukotriene receptor antagonist ICI 204,219 on allergen-induced bronchoconstriction and airway hyperreactivity in atopic subjects. Lancet. 1991; 337: 690–4.

15. Rasmussen JB, Eriksson L-O, Margolskee DJ, Tagari P, Williams VC, Andersson K-E. Leukotriene D_4 receptor blocker inhibits the immediate and late bronchoconstrictor responses to inhaled antigen in patients with asthma. J Allergy Clin Immunol. 1992; 90: 193–201.

16. Kane GC, Pollice M, Kim C-J, et al. A controlled trial of the effect of the 5-lipoxygenase inhibitor, zileuton, on lung inflammation produced by segmental antigen challenge in human beings. J Allergy Clin Immunol. 1996; 97: 646–54.

17. Wenzel SE, Trudeau JB, Kaminsky DA, Cohn J, Martin RJ, Westcott JY. Effect of 5-lipoxygenase inhibition on bronchoconstriction and airway inflammation in nocturnal asthma. Am J Resp Crit Care Med. 1995; 152: 897–905.

18. Calhoun WJ, Williams KL, Simonson SG, Lavins BJ. Effect of zafirlukast (Accolate™) on airway inflammation after segmental allergen challenge in patients with mild asthma. Am J Respir Crit Care Med. 1997; 155: A662.

19. Leff JA, Pizzichini E, Efthimiadis A, et al. Effect of montelukast (MK-0476) on airway eosinophilic inflammation in mildly uncontrolled asthma: A randomized placebo-controlled trial. Am J Resp Crit Care Med. 1997; 155: A977.

20. Liu MC, Dube LM, Lancaster J, Zileuton Study Group. Acute and chronic effects of a 5-lipoxygenase inhibitor in asthma: A 6-month randomized multicenter trial. J Allergy Clin Immunol. 1996; 98: 859–71.

21. Calhoun WJ, Weisberg SC, Faiferman I, Stober PW. Pranlukast (Ultair™) is effective

in improving asthma: results of a 12-week, multicenter, dose-ranging study. J Allergy Clin Immunol. 1997; 99: S318.

22. Spector SL, Smith LJ, Glass M. Effect of 6 weeks of therapy with oral doses of ICI 204,219, a leukotriene D_4 receptor antagonist, in subjects with bronchial asthma. Am J Resp Crit Care Med. 1994; 150: 618–23.

23. Tashkin DP, Nelson HS, Cohn J, Hanby LA, Miller CJ. Efficacy and safety of zafirlukast (Accolate) in patients with mild to moderate asthma. Am J Resp Crit Care Med. 1996; 153: A534.

24. Suissa S, Dennis R, Ernst P, Sheehy O, Wooddauphine. Effectiveness of the leukotriene receptor antagonist zafirlukast for mild-to-moderate asthma – a randomized double-blind, placebo-controlled trial. Ann Intern Med. 1997; 126: 177.

25. Reiss TF, Chervinsky P, Edwards T, et al. Montelukast Study Group. Montelukast (MK-0476), a Cys LT_1 receptor antagonist, improves asthma outcomes over a 3-month treatment period. Am J Resp Crit Care Med. 1997; 155: A662.

26. Sahn S, Galant S, Murray J, et al., on behalf of the Ultair Study Group. Pranlukast (Ultair™) improves FEV_1 in patients with asthma: results of a 12-week multicenter study vs Nedocromil. Am J Resp Crit Care Med. 1997; 155: A665.

27. Nathan RA, Glass M, Snader L. Effects of 13 weeks of treatment with ICI 204,219 (Accolate™) or cromolyn sodium (Intal™) in patients with mild to moderate asthma. J Allergy Clin Immunol. 1995; 95: S388.

28. Wenzel P, Chervinsky P, Kerwin E, Silvers W, Faiferman I, Dubb J. Oral pranlukast (Ultair™) vs inhaled beclomethasone: Results of a 12-week trial in patients with asthma. Am J Resp Crit Care Med. 1997; 155: A203.

29. Tamaoki J, Kondo M, Sakai N, et al. Leukotriene antagonist prevents exacerbation of asthma during reduction of high-dose inhaled corticosteroid. Am J Resp Crit Care Med. 1997; 155: 1235–40.

30. Bateman ED, Holgate ST, Binks SM, Tams IP. A multicenter study to assess the steroid-sparing potential of Accolate™ (Zafirlukast; 20mg BD). Allergy. 1995; 50: P-0709.

31. Laitinin LA, Zetterstrom O, Holgate ST, Binks SM, Whitney JG. Effects of Accolate™ (Zafirlukast; 20mg BD) in permitting reduced therapy with inhaled steroids: a multicenter trial in patients with doses of inhaled steroid optimised between 800 and 2000 mcg per day. Allergy. 1995; 50: P-0710.

32. O'Connor BJ, Godard P, Dube LM, Swanson LJ, Rountree LV. The effect of 5-lipoxygenase inhibitor, zileuton, plus low-dose inhaled beclomethasone compared to higher dose beclomethasone alone in patients with asthma. Am J Resp Crit Care Med. 1996; 153: A803.

33. Christie PE, Tagari P, Ford-Hutchinson AW, et al. Urinary leukotriene E_4 concentrations increase after aspirin challenge in aspirin sensitive asthmatic subjects. Am Rev Resp Dis. 1991; 143: 1025–9.

34. Arm JS, O'Hickey S, Spur BW, Lee TH. Airway responsiveness to histamine and leukotriene E_4 in subjects with aspirin-induced asthma. Am Rev Resp Dis. 1987; 140: 148–53.

35. Dahlén B, Margolskee DJ, Zetterstrom O, Dahlén S-E. Effect of the leukotriene receptor antagonist MK-0679 on baseline pulmonary function in aspirin sensitive asthmatic subjects. Thorax. 1993; 48: 1205–10.

36. Israel E, Fischer AR, Rosenberg MA, et al. The pivotal role of 5-lipoxygenase products in the reaction of aspirin-sensitive asthmatics to aspirin. Am Rev Resp Dis. 1993; 148: 1447–51.

37. Kuna P, Malmstrom K, Dahlén S-E, et al. Montelukast (MK-0476), a $CysLT_1$ antagonist, improves asthma control in aspirin-intolerant asthmatic patients. Am J Resp Crit Care Med. 1997; 155: A975.

38. The British Guidelines on asthma management 1995. Review and position statement. Thorax. 1997; 52: S1–21.

39. Guidelines for the diagnosis and management of asthma. Bethesda, MD: National Institutes of Health. February 1997.

11 Transcription factors HSF and NF-κB as targets for cytoprotective eicosanoids: a new strategy for therapeutic intervention

M. G. SANTORO

The observation that an increase in temperature of a few degrees above the physiological level induces the synthesis of a small number of proteins in *Drosophila* salivary glands led to the discovery of a universal protective mechanism which prokaryotic and eukaryotic cells utilize to preserve cellular function and homeostasis[1]. This complex physiological defence mechanism, known as the heat shock response, involves the rapid induction of a specific set of genes encoding cytoprotective proteins (heat shock protein, HSP). In mammalian cells HSP synthesis is induced in a wide variety of toxic conditions, including extreme temperatures, oxidative stress, exposure to heavy metals or cytotoxic drugs, glucose deprivation and virus infection[1]. Whereas HSP induction was at first interpreted as a signal for detection of physiological stress, it is now well-documented that HSPs are utilized by the cells in the repair process following different types of injury, to prevent damage resulting from the accumulation and aggregation of non-native proteins[2].

Induction requires the activation and translocation to the nucleus of a transregulatory protein, the heat shock transcription factor (HSF). In mammalian cells, HSF exists as an inactive non-DNA binding form, which is rapidly converted to the DNA-binding form upon exposure to heat shock or other stimuli[3]. HSF activation is a multistep process and requires oligomerization, acquisition of DNA-binding activity, localization to the nucleus and phosphorylation by an as yet unknown kinase[3]. In the nucleus HSF binds to specific promoter elements (HSE) located upstream of heat shock (*hs*) genes, activating transcription. Several HSFs (HSF1–HSF4) have been identified in vertebrate cells [3]; however, the molecular mechanisms responsible for signal transduction which leads to HSF activation and phosphorylation have not been completely elucidated.

HSP can be divided into five families, depending on their molecular weight. In eukaryotic cells 70 kDa heat shock proteins (hsp 70), which are encoded by a large multigene family, include the constitutively expressed hsc70, the major inducible hsp70, the inducible hsp72, the glucose regulated grp78/BiP and the mitochondrial P75[3]. In mammalian cells, several HSP that function as molecular chaperones and are essential for a correct folding, assembly and intracellular translocation of proteins, are expressed during normal growth conditions and can be induced by biologically active molecules such as haemin[4] and prostaglandins[5].

CYTOPROTECTIVE ROLE OF HEAT SHOCK PROTEINS IN HUMAN DISEASES

In the last few years, the cytoprotective role of HSP has been described in several human diseases, including metabolic disorders[6], inflammation[7], infection[8] and ischaemia[9]. In cardiac tissues a wide variety of insults, including myocardial ischaemia, trauma and hyperthermia, results in the synthesis of HSP, which have been shown to play a pivotal role in restoring normal cardiac function after injury, possibly by removal of denatured cardiac proteins and re-establishment of normal cardiac protein synthesis. A correlation has been shown between the amount of hsp70 and the degree of myocardial protection in vitro as well as in animal models[9,10]. Moreover, transfected heart-derived cells overexpressing hsp70 and hsp70-transgenic mice show enhanced resistance to ischaemic stress, providing evidence for a direct role of this protein in cytoprotection after this type of injury[9,11]. A pharmacological approach to hsp70 induction and cardiac protection is suggested by the recently described hsp70-induced protection by simulated ischaemia in rat neonatal cardiomyocytes treated with the hsp70 inducer herbimycin-A[12]. In the case of inflammation, HSP have been shown to protect mammalian cells from tumour necrosis factors α- and β-mediated cytotoxicity[13], as well as to suppress astroglial-inducible nitric oxide synthase expression[14]. Moreover, in a rodent model for adult respiratory distress syndrome (ARDS), pre-exposure of animals to heat shock, leading to massive induction of hsp70 within

Figure 1 **Activation of the heat-shock response and inhibition of NF-κB by cyclopentenone prostaglandins. (A) Synthesis of cytoprotective heat-shock proteins is induced by PG via the activation of heat-shock transcription factor HSF. HSF converts from a monomeric non-DNA-binding form to an oligomeric form that translocates to the nucleus and binds to specific promoter elements (HSE) located upstream of heat-shock genes (e.g. HSP70). (B) Effect of arachidonic acid metabolites on HSF activation. Whole-cell extracts of Jurkat cells treated with 24 μM arachidonic acid (AA), PGA$_1$, PGB$_1$, PGD$_2$, PGE$_1$, PGF$_2\alpha$ or diluent control (c) for 6 h were incubated with a ^{32}P-labelled HSE probe, followed by analysis of DNA-binding activity by EMSA (21). Position of HSF-DNA binding complex (HSF), constitutive HSE-binding activity (CHBA) and non-specific protein –DNA interactions (NS) are shown. (C) Inhibition of NF-κB activation. NF-κB normally exists in an inactive cytoplasmic complex, whose predominant form is a heterodimer composed of p50 and p65 subunits, bound to the inhibitory protein IκBα. Cyclopentenone prostaglandins act by inhibiting IκBα phosphorylation and degradation. (D) Whole-cell extracts from Jurkat cells treated with AA, PGA$_1$, PGB$_1$, PGD$_2$, PGE$_1$, PGF$_2\alpha$ or diluent control (c) for 2 h and then stimulated with 12-O-tetradecanoylphorbol 13-acetate (TPA) for 6 h were incubated with a ^{32}P-labelled κB DNA probe, followed by EMSA. Position of NF-κB-DNA complex (NF-κB) and non-specific binding (ns) are indicated. Control cells are neither stimulated with TPA nor treated with prostaglandins**

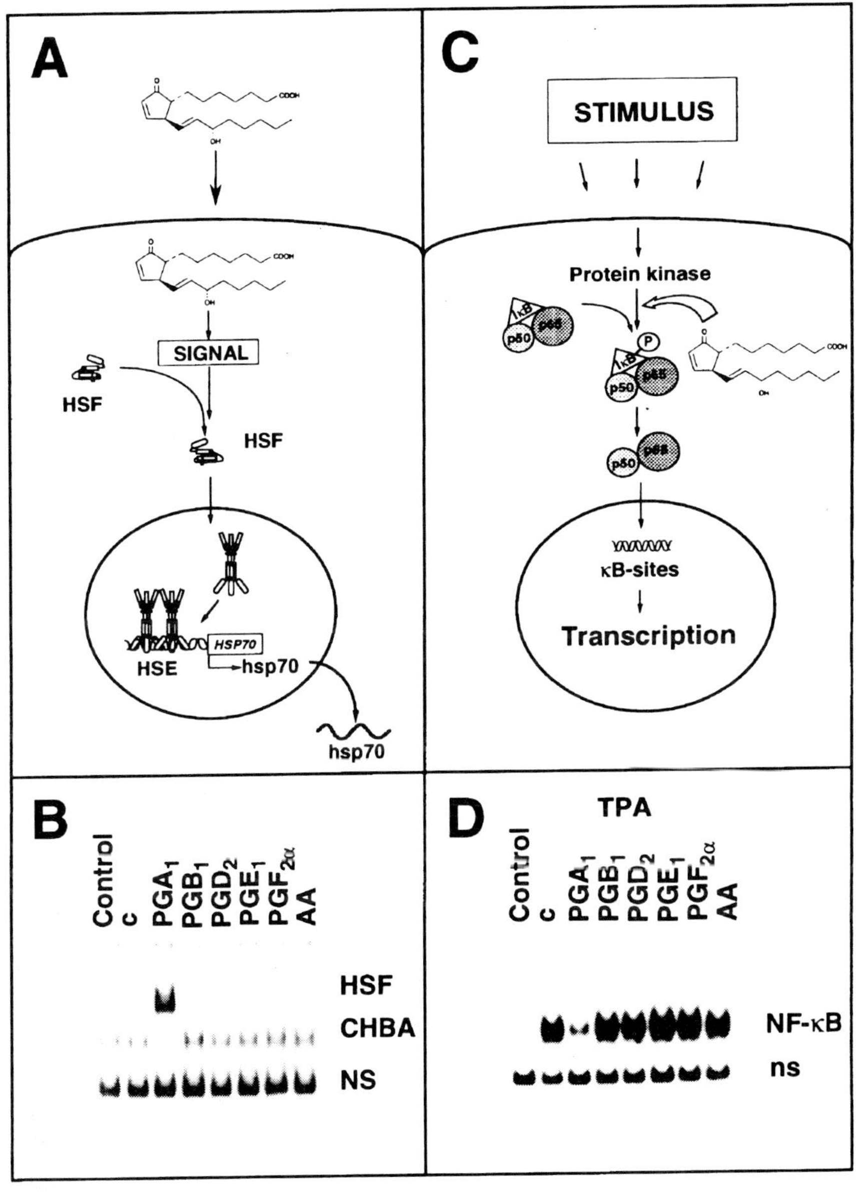
A
SIGNAL
HSF
HSF
HSP70
HSE
hsp70
hsp70
C
STIMULUS
Protein kinase
κB
p50
p65
P
κB
p50
p65
p50
p65
κB-sites
Transcription
B
Control
c
PGA1
PGB1
PGD2
PGE1
PGF2α
AA
HSF
CHBA
NS
D
TPA
Control
c
PGA1
PGB1
PGD2
PGE1
PGF2α
AA
NF-κB
ns

the lung, is associated with decreased pulmonary inflammation and prevention of death[15]. Increased expression of hsp70 has also been associated with inhibition of virus replication during acute infection[8,16]. These observations suggest new therapeutic strategies relying upon the development of drugs which selectively turn on heat shock genes.

EICOSANOIDS AND THE HEAT SHOCK RESPONSE

We have shown that cyclooxygenase cyclopentenone metabolites such as prostaglandins of the A and J type (PGAs and PGJs) induce the synthesis of hsp70 in a non-stressful situation in a wide variety of human and mammalian cells (reviewed in 17,18), whereas leukotrienes, and in particular LTB_4, do not activate HSF nor stimulate HSP expression in human and murine cells (Elia G, Santoro MG, unpublished results). The mechanism of hsp70 induction by cyclopentenone prostaglandins via cycloheximide-sensitive activation of HSF1 (Figure 1) and the kinetics of *hsp70* gene transcription and hsp70 protein synthesis have been well characterized in human cells[19]. The PGJ metabolite 15-deoxy-$\Delta^{12,14}$PGJ$_2$, which was shown to be the natural ligand for the adipocyte determination factor PPARγ inducing adipocyte differentiation[20], is also a potent inducer of HSF activation[21]. We have also shown that PGA_1 and PGJ_2 induce the synthesis of the oxidative stress protein haeme oxygenase in murine myoblasts[22] and in human monocytes from healthy donors (Elia et al., in preparation). Structure–activity relationship studies have recently shown that HSP induction requires the presence of a reactive α,β-unsaturated carbonyl group in the cyclopentane ring (cyclopentenone), which renders this portion of the molecule able to form Michael's adducts with cellular nucleophilics, and to covalently bind to cysteine residues of proteins[23].

Induction of hsp70 by cyclopentenone prostaglandins is associated with a cytoprotective effect during hyperthermia and virus infection: cyclopentenone prostaglandins induce a thermotolerant state in human cells and protect cells from subsequent lethal injury[24]. Cyclopentenone prostaglandins are also characterized by a potent antiviral activity against a wide variety of DNA and RNA viruses, including the human immunodeficiency virus (HIV-1), in several experimental models in vitro and in vivo (reviewed in 25). A long-acting synthetic analogue of PGA_2 (di-M-PGA$_2$) has antiviral activity in a mouse model infected with influenza A virus[26]. In negative strand RNA virus models prostaglandins of the A and J type provoke a selective and dramatic block of viral protein synthesis[8,27]. This block is exerted at the translational level and is dependent on hsp70 expression in infected cells. A possible model has been hypothesized in which HSP and virus messages, both of which can be translated in conditions where cellular protein synthesis is impaired, could possess similar mechanisms for preferential translation, and could then compete with each other[25]. In the case of HIV-1 infection, a single treatment with PGA_1 or PGJ_2 is cytoprotective in lymphoblastoid CEM-SS cells, and causes a more than 1000-fold reduction in infectious virus yield, due to a selective block of HIV-1 mRNA transcription[28]. Inhibition of HIV-1 RNA transcription appears to be mediated by the recently discovered ability of cyclopentenone PGs to inhibit the activation of nuclear factor-κB (NF-κB)[21].

NUCLEAR FACTOR κ-B

NF-κB is an inducible eukaryotic transcription factor of the *rel* family, which normally exists in an inactive cytoplasmic complex, whose predominant form is a heterodimer composed of p50 and p65 (Rel A) subunits, bound to inhibitory proteins of the IκB family, usually IκBα, and is activated in response to primary (viruses, bacteria, UV) or secondary (inflammatory cytokines) pathogenic stimuli[29,30]. Stimulation triggers rapid phosphorylation and degradation of IκBα, resulting in NF-κB translocation to the nucleus, where it binds to DNA at specific κB-sites, rapidly inducing a variety of genes encoding signalling proteins. Target genes include cyclooxygenase-2, nitric-oxide synthase (iNOS), several inflammatory and chemotactic cytokines, cytokine receptors, cell adhesion molecules as well as viral genes[29]. NF-κB is a critical regulator of the immediate early pathogen response and activation of the immune system, and is involved in many pathological events, including progression of AIDS by enhancing HIV-1 transcription[31]. A possible role for NF-κB in atherosclerosis and reoxygenation damage has also been suggested[32,33]. Consequently NF-κB is an attractive therapeutic target for novel anti-inflammatory, antiviral and cytoprotective drugs, and the need for the development of effective NF-κB inhibitors with therapeutic efficacy is widely recognized.

Several arachidonic acid metabolites appear to interfere with NF-κB activation. 12(R)-hydroxyeicosatrienoic acid [12(R)-HETrE], but not the enantiomer 12(S)-HETrE, was found to markedly activate NF-κB DNA-binding activity in coronary microvessel endothelial cells[34]. 5-Lipoxygenase inhibitors (nordihydroguaiaretic acid and AA861), but not cyclooxygenase inhibitors, were reported to block IL-1β-induced expression of cell surface adhesion molecules (VCAM-1), via inhibition of NF-κB in human cells[35]. Leukotriene B_4 was also reported to activate NF-κB and NF-κB-controlled interleukin-6 expression in human blood monocytes[36]. However, we were unable to detect any significant increase in the constitutive level of DNA-binding activity of NF-κB in human peripheral blood monocytes in the presence of concentrations of LTB_4 ranging from 10^{-11} to 10^{-6} M (Elia G, Santoro MG, unpublished data). On the other hand, we have recently reported that cyclopentenone prostaglandins are potent inhibitors of NF-κB activation in human cells, and of NF-κB-dependent HIV-1 transcription in long terminal repeat-chloramphenicol acetyl transferase transient transfection experiments[21]. These eicosanoids act by inhibiting phosphorylation and preventing degradation of the NF-κB inhibitor IκBα[21]. Inhibition does not require protein synthesis and is dependent on the presence of a reactive cyclopentenonic moiety. Interestingly, the NF-κB inhibitory effect is tightly associated with HSF activation in human cells[21]. In fact activation of HSF1 by different cyclopentenone prostaglandins, by other chemical inducers, such as sodium arsenite, or by hyperthermia itself was found to prevent or suppress NF-κB activation, indicating a link between the regulatory pathways of these factors and suggesting the possibility that triggering of HSF1 could render cells unresponsive to stimulation of NF-κB. This hypothesis is very attractive considering the opposite roles of HSF and NF-κB in cytoprotection and cell injury respectively, as in the case of inflammation[14] and viral infection[8, 25, 31] (Figure 2).

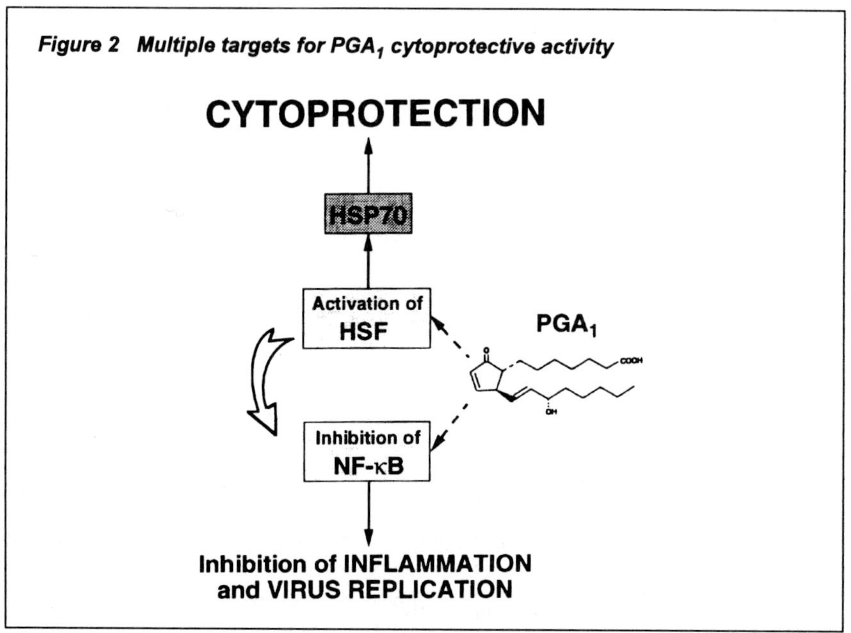

PERSPECTIVES AND CONCLUSIONS

These observations encourage the search for novel prostanoids with the ability to induce HSP and inhibit NF-κB simultaneously, which could be utilized as cytoprotective and antiviral drugs. Prostaglandins are used clinically in the treatment of several diseases, including gastric ulcers and congenital heart disease, and to facilitate labour, and are generally effective and well-tolerated[37]. Administration of PGE_1 has also been shown to be beneficial in patients with fulminant viral hepatitis[38]. In studies on volunteers with hypertension, infusion with PGA_1 had beneficial effects on blood pressure, while no deleterious effects on kidney function or other significant side-effects were found[39]. On the other hand, the fact that different types of PGs are synthesized in different tissues throughout the body and have multiple effects on blood pressure, inflammatory and immune responses, poses several questions on the possible use of natural prostaglandins as cytoprotective compounds.

We have recently reported that one component of the PGA molecule, 2-cyclopenten-1-one, is able to activate HSF and to trigger rapid and selective transcription and translation of the *hsp70* gene, leading to the accumulation of high levels of hsp70 protein in human cells[23]. As previously shown for other HSP inducers, including antiviral prostaglandins, sodium arsenite, cadmium and hyperthermia itself, 2-cyclopenten-1-one-induced hsp70 synthesis is associated with a selective inhibition of virus protein synthesis, and viral replication[23]. The α,β-unsaturated carbonyl group present in 2-cyclopenten-1-one is the molecular structure responsible for HSF activation, since even high concentrations of cyclopentanone (a similar molecule with a saturated carbonyl), or cyclopentene, which contains a double bond, but not a carbonyl group were unable to induce HSF DNA-binding activity. These results indicate that a class of novel molecules, characterized by the ability to activate HSF while inhibiting NF-κB, and devoid of the pleiotropic effects of natural PGs could be designed, opening new perspectives for therapeutic intervention in inflammatory and infectious diseases.

Acknowledgements

This work was supported by a grant from the Italian Ministry of Public Health, 1997 AIDS Research project and Multiple Sclerosis project, and CNR P.S. 'Stress Proteins'.

References

1. Linquist S, Craig EA. The heat shock proteins. Annu Rev Genet. 1988; 22: 631–77.
2. Feige U, Morimoto RI, Yahara I, Polla BS. Stress-Inducible Cellular Responses. Basel–Boston–Berlin: Birkhäuser-Verlag, 1996.
3. Morimoto RI, Sarge KD, Abravaya K. Transcriptional regulation of heat shock genes. J Biol Chem. 1992; 267: 21987–90.
4. Sistonen L, Sarge KD, Phillips B, Abravaya K, Morimoto RI. Activation of heat shock factor 2 during hemin-induced differentiation of human erythroleukemia cells. Mol Cell Biol. 1992; 12: 4104–11.
5. Santoro MG, Garaci E, Amici C. Prostaglandins with antiproliferative activity induce the synthesis of a heat shock protein in human cells. Proc Natl Acad Sci USA. 1989; 86: 8407–11.
6. Williams RS, Thomas JA, Fina M, German Z, Benjamin IJ. Human heat shock protein 70 (hsp70) protects murine cells from injury during metabolic stress. J Clin Invest. 1993; 92: 503–8.
7. Polla BS, Cossarizza A. Stress proteins in inflammation. In: Feige U, Morimoto RI, Yahara I, Polla BS, editors. Stress-Inducible Cellular Responses. Basel–Boston–Berlin: Birkhäuser-Verlag, 1996: 375–91.
8. Amici C, Giorgi C, Rossi A, Santoro MG. Selective inhibition of virus protein synthesis by prostaglandin A: A translational block associated with HSP70 synthesis. J Virol. 1994; 68: 6890–9.
9. Mestril R, Chi SH, Sayen MR, O'Reilly K, Dillmann WH. Expression of inducible stress protein 70 in rat heart myogenic cells confers protection against stimulated ischemia-induced injury. J Clin Invest. 1994; 93: 759–67.
10. Marber MS, Walker JM, Latchman DS, Yellon DM. Myocardial protection after whole body heat stress in the rabbit is dependent on metabolic substrate and is related to the amount of the inducible 70-KD heat stress protein. J Clin Invest. 1994; 93: 1087–94.
11. Plumier J, Ross BM, Currie RW, et al. Transgenic mice expressing the human heat shock protein 70 have improved post-ischemic myocardial recovery. J Clin Invest. 1995; 95: 1854–60.
12. Morris SD, Cumming DV, Latchman DS, Yellon DM. Specific induction of the 70-kD heat stress protein by the tyrosine kinase inhibitor herbimycin-A protects rat neonatal cardiomyocytes. J Clin Invest. 1996; 97: 706–12.
13. Iaattela M, Wissing D, Bauer PA, Li GC. Major heat shock protein hsp70 protects tumor cells from tumor necrosis factor cytotoxicity. EMBO J. 1992; 11: 3507–12.
14. Feinstein DL, Galea E, Aquino DA, Li GC, Xu H, Reis DJ. Heat shock protein 70 suppresses astroglial-inducible nitric-oxide synthase expression by decreasing NF-κB activation. J Biol Chem. 1996; 271: 17724–32.
15. Villar J, Edelson JD, Post M, Brendan J, Mullen M, Slutsky AS. Induction of heat stress proteins is associated with decreased mortality in an animal model of acute lung injury. Am Rev Resp Dis. 1993; 147: 177–81.
16. Santoro MG. Viral infection. In: Feige U, Morimoto RI, Yahara I, Polla BS, editors. Stress-Inducible Cellular Responses. Basel–Boston–Berlin: Birkhäuser-Verlag, 1996: 337–57.

17. Santoro MG, Garaci E, Amici C. Induction of HSP70 by prostaglandins. In: Schlesinger MJ, Santoro MG, Garaci E, editors. Stress Proteins: Induction and Function. Berlin: Springer-Verlag, 1990: 27–44.

18. Santoro MG. Heat shock proteins and virus replication: Hsp70s as mediators of the antiviral effects of prostaglandins. Experientia. 1994; 50: 1039–47.

19. Amici C, Sistonen L, Santoro MG, Morimoto RI. Antiproliferative prostaglandins activate heat shock transcription factor. Proc Natl Acad Sci USA. 1992; 89: 6227–31.

20. Kliewer SA, Lenhard JM, Wilson TM, Patel I, Morris DC, Lehmann JM. A prostaglandin J_2 metabolite binds peroxisome proliferator-activated receptor γ and promotes adipocyte differentiation. Cell 1995; 83: 813–19.

21. Rossi A, Elia G, Santoro MG. Inhibition of nuclear factor κB by prostaglandin A_1: An effect associated with heat shock transcription factor activation. Proc Natl Acad Sci USA. 1997; 94: 746–50.

22. Rossi A, Santoro MG. Induction by prostaglandin A_1 of haem oxygenase in myoblastic cells: An effect independent of expression of the 70 kDa heat shock protein. Biochem J. 1995; 308: 455–63.

23. Rossi A, Elia G, Santoro MG. 2-Cyclopenten-1-one, a new inducer of heat shock protein 70 with antiviral activity. J Biol Chem. 1996; 271: 32192–6.

24. Amici C, Palamara AT, Santoro MG. Induction of thermotolerance by prostaglandin A in human cells. Exp Cell Res. 1993; 207: 230–4.

25. Santoro MG. Antiviral activity of cyclopentenone prostanoids. Trends Microbiol. 1997; 5: 276–81.

26. Santoro MG, Favalli C, Mastino A, Jaffe BM, Esteban M, Garaci E. Antiviral activity of a synthetic analog of prostaglandin A in mice infected with influenza A virus. Arch Virol. 1988; 99: 89–100.

27. Pica F, De Marco A, De Cesare F, Santoro MG. Inhibition of vesicular stomatitis virus replication by Δ^{12}-prostaglandin J_2 is regulated at two separate levels and is associated with induction of stress protein synthesis. Antiviral Res. 1993; 20: 193–208.

28. Rozera C, Carattoli A, De Marco A, Amici C, Giorgi C, Santoro MG. Inhibition of HIV-1 replication by cyclopentenone prostaglandins in acutely infected human cells. J Clin Invest. 1996; 97: 1795–803.

29. Baldwin AS. The NF-κB and IκB proteins: New discoveries and insights. Annu Rev Immunol. 1996; 14: 649–81.

30. Bauerle PA, Baltimore D. NF-κB: Ten years after. Cell. 1996; 87: 13–20.

31. Nabel G, Baltimore D. An inducible transcription factor activates expression of human immunodeficiency virus in T cells. Nature. 1987; 326: 711–13.

32. Brand K, Page S, Rogler G, et al. Activated transcription factor nuclear factor-kappa B is present in the atherosclerotic lesion. J Clin Invest. 1996; 97: 1715–22.

33. Rupec RA, Baeuerle PA. The genomic response of tumor cells to hypoxia and reoxygenation. Differential activation of transcription factors AP-1 and NF-κB. Eur J Biochem. 1995; 234: 632–40.

34. Stoltz RA, Abraham NG, Laniado-Schwartzman M. The role of NF-kappa B in the angiogenic response of coronary microvessel endothelial cells. Proc Natl Acad Sci USA. 1996; 93: 2832–7.

35. Lee S, Felts KA, Parry GC, Armacost LM, Cobb RR. Inhibition of 5-lipoxygenase blocks IL-1 beta-induced vascular adhesion molecule-1 gene expression in human endothelial cells. J Immunol. 1997; 158: 3401–7.

36. Brach MA, de Vos S, Arnold C, Gruß HJ, Mertelsmann R, Herrmann F. Leukotriene B_4 transcriptionally activates interleukin-6 expression involving NF-κB and NF-IL6. Eur J Immunol. 1992; 22: 2705–11.

37. Shield MJ. Novel applications of misoprostol. Pharmacol Ther. 1995; 65: 125–47.

38. Sinclair SB, Greig PD, Blendis LM, et al. Biochemical and clinical response of fulminant viral hepatitis to administration of prostaglandin E. J Clin Invest. 1989; 84: 1063–9.

39. Lee J, Kannegiesser H, O'Toole J, Westura E. Hypertension and the renomedullary prostaglandins: A human study of the antihypertensive effects of PGA_1. Ann NY Acad Sci. 1971; 180: 218–40.

12 Vascular biology of the leukotrienes

J.-P. GASCARD and C. BRINK

While the mechanisms responsible for asthma have not been identified, many of the respiratory measurements and symptoms have led physicians to accept the hypothesis that this disease has an allergic component. In clinical trials used to establish the efficacy of potentially new therapeutic drugs, a protocol involving allergen inhalation is frequently performed in asthmatic subjects. The ability of the compound to effectively block the bronchoconstriction or limit the severity of the allergen challenge is taken as an initial sign that the drug may have some therapeutic value in asthma. However, the hallmarks of extreme anaphylactic reactions are not only dyspnoea but also severe hypotension. Milder allergic inflammatory responses are associated with increased blood flow, extravasation of plasma and the recruitment of circulating leukocytes into the tissue compartment. Thus a cardinal sign of activation of inflammatory cells by allergen is a marked alteration in vascular tone and reactivity. These vascular modifications may also contribute to those effects observed in asthmatic patients subsequent to allergen inhalation.

The problem is how to evaluate release of cysteinyl-leukotrienes (cys-LTs) in the human pulmonary circulation either during allergen inhalation or under other clinical conditions. In this presentation, the results are based on a cardiovascular surgical intervention, during which the release of cys-LTs from the human lung and the capacity of these mediators to modify pulmonary vascular tone were monitored.

ALLERGEN CHALLENGE IN THE HUMAN LUNG

Schild and co-workers[1] demonstrated that human lung from asthmatic patients released slow reacting substance of anaphylaxis (SRS-A) when stimulated with an appropriate antigen. Confirmation of this initial observation was provided by the work of Brocklehurst[2] and Dahlén and co-workers[3]. Reports based on human lung tissues passively sensitized[4,5] and then challenged with antigen provided further evidence that tissues from the human lung produced and released these potent mediators. Since the original description of SRS-A, this entity is now known[6] to be a composite of leukotrienes (LTC_4, LTD_4 and LTE_4).

Circumstantial evidence in support of the concept that these mediators may play a pivotal role in airway disease such as asthma was derived from the clinical observations that several cell types that produce cys-LTs (mast cells, basophils and eosinophils) are present in increased numbers in the lungs of asthmatic patients. In addition, the detection of these metabolites in biological fluids from asthmatic subjects following allergen provocation in clinical studies further supported this concept. Lam and co-workers[7] detected LTC_4 and LTB_4 in sputum obtained from asthmatic patients. However, these investigators were unable to measure the 5-lipoxygenase (5-LO) metabolites in sputum from patients with other lung diseases. Taylor and co-workers[8] measured urinary LTE_4 levels and reported an elevated level in asthmatic patients following antigen inhalation. These observations have been confirmed by a number of other investigators and demonstrate the release of cys-LTs in asthmatic patients. However, whether or not the human lung in vivo is responsible or associated with this release in asthmatic patients is presently unknown.

RELEASE OF CYSTEINYL-LEUKOTRIENES BY HUMAN LUNG IN SITU

The implication that metabolites of the arachidonic acid cascade, specifically products of the 5-LO pathway, may be released from the human lung in asthma or in vascular disease such as pulmonary hypertension has been supported by measurement of these metabolites in peripheral blood samples[9], urine[10] and bronchoalveolar lavage fluid[11,12]. The results of these studies provide only indirect evidence of cys-LT release from the lung and interpretation is difficult since the quantities detected in the peripheral blood and urine may reflect more than simply lung production and/or release. Furthermore, in adult asthmatics attempts to measure cys-LTs in plasma suggested that the levels are often undetectable in both normal and asthmatic subjects.

A number of surgical reports have shown acute transitory episodes of increased pulmonary arterial pressure in patients following open heart surgery for correction of congenital heart lesions[13]. During surgery the lung is subjected to a period of reperfusion, an event which may provoke mediator release and cause vasospasm. Under such conditions the released mediators may account for the transitory increases in pulmonary arterial pressure that are frequently observed in infants. Since the circulating levels of cys-LTs in infants with congenital heart defects are not known, the levels of LTE_4 in blood samples from patients with increased pulmonary blood flow and pulmonary hypertension (PH) were determined during the surgical intervention for correction of the heart defect and compared with infants with decreased pulmonary blood flow (control). Eighteen patients with congenital heart defects (<25 months of age) were studied. Six were diagnosed to have the regular form of tetralogy of Fallot (control), seven patients had complete atrioventricular septal defect, three had truncus arteriosus and two had ventricular septal defect. All patients with PH (n = 12) presented with heart failure despite medical therapy support. None received medication that could interfere with the arachidonic acid cascade. Haemodynamic measurements (pulmonary, systemic and atrial pressures) were continuously recorded for each patient using a Hewlet Packard 78354A monitor. After sternal and pericardial opening, blood samples were drawn from the main pulmonary artery and the left atrium at different times during the surgical intervention. Blood samples were collected at the beginning of extracorporeal circulation (ECC), 5 minutes after lung reperfusion and at the end of ECC. The samples were collected directly into tubes containing methanol and stored at –20°C overnight. They were then thawed, vortexed and centrifuged (5000 rpm for 20 minutes at 4°C). The supernatant was removed and added to tubes containing 40 ml of methanol at 10% and this mixture was then passed through a column (Sep-Pak C-18). The extracts containing lipids were collected on 3 ml of methanol and then separated into equal volume aliquots and dried using a Speed-Vac evaporator. The residue was dissolved in mobile phase solution of HPLC (acetonitrile/water/acetic acid at pH 5.6). This solution (20 μl) was injected into an HPLC (Waters) for separation. The samples were collected and quantification was performed by an enzyme immunoassay (EIA).

The LTE_4 levels detected in the infants during the course of the surgical intervention are shown in Table 1. In five of the 18 patients examined (one Fallot, four PH), LTE_4 levels were below the threshold level of detection. In the two groups of patients the total quantities of LTE_4 detected during the surgical intervention were similar. An increase in the circulating LTE_4 blood levels was not observed in those patients with pulmonary hypertension. These data, derived from a limited number of patients, suggested that the circulating LTE_4 blood levels remained constant during the surgical intervention. However, there was considerable variation in the LTE_4 levels detected in blood samples obtained from neonates with or without pulmonary hypertension. The range in the quantities of LTE_4 detected were similar to those reported by other investigators when this metabolite was measured in either urine[10], bronchoalveolar lavage[11] or blood samples[9] from patients with different clinical pathologies. The reasons for these variations are unknown but may be independent of the pathophysiological condition, since both control subjects (Fallot) as well as infants with PH exhibited a considerable range in LTE_4 values: 0–0.76 ng/ml blood and 0–7.2 ng/ml blood, respectively.

Table 1 Detection of LTE_4 in blood samples from infants

Condition	Peripheral blood (ng/ml of blood)	ECC total (ng/ml of blood)
Fallot ($n = 6$)	0.44±0.12 (6)	0.64±0.17(35)
Pulmonary hypertension ($n = 12$)	1.37±0.67(12)	1.03±0.44(67)

ECC, Extracorporeal circulation.
Values are means ± SEM. Numbers in parentheses are the number of measurements performed.

CYSTEINYL-LEUKOTRIENE EFFECTS IN THE PULMONARY VASCULAR BED IN VITRO

A considerable amount of information is available concerning the contractile properties of cysteinyl-leukotrienes (cys-LT) on smooth muscle. However, only a limited amount of data is available on the effects of these mediators in the pulmonary vascular bed in vivo. Injection of LTD_4 caused a significant increase of pulmonary arterial pressure in the guinea-pig[14]. In addition, Gause and co-workers[15] demonstrated that the pulmonary arterial pressure was elevated in utero in lambs and that this elevated pressure was reduced significantly after a bolus injection of FPL 55712. These results suggested that cys-LTs may be associated with elevated pulmonary pressure. However,

Secrest and co-workers[16] reported that in canine renal arteries LTD_4 induced relaxations which were produced by stimulation of a receptor since they were attenuated by FPL 55712. These investigators further showed that LTD_4 also increased cGMP accumulation in canine vessels[17]. Together these observations indicated the presence of leukotriene receptors on the endothelium and suggested that the relaxations may be via the liberation of nitric oxide. Initial studies by Sukuma and Levi[18] demonstrated that pulmonary arteries from the guinea-pig also relaxed when stimulated by LTD_4. No attempt was made by these authors to explore the receptors or the mechanisms involved in the relaxations. These data clearly demonstrated that the cys-LTs exhibited paradoxical effects (contraction/relaxation) in vessels derived from a number of vascular beds in different species. In human isolated pulmonary vessels, Ortiz and co-workers[19] characterized and localized the cys-LT receptors. A brief résumé of these results (Figure 1) has recently been published[20]. These results demonstrated the presence of two cys-LT receptors on the endothelium of human pulmonary veins. One receptor ($CysLT_1$) when stimulated by LTD_4 is associated with the release of a contractile factor. This contraction was blocked by $CysLT_1$ antagonists. A second receptor ($CysLT_2$) found on the endothelium of the pulmonary vasculature which when stimulated by LTD_4 caused the release of nitric oxide. This receptor was resis tant to the classical $CysLT_1$ antagonists. In addition, the $CysLT_2$ receptor[21] is also present on the vascular smooth muscle and stimulation of this receptor is associated with contraction. Whether or not the $CysLT_2$ receptor on the endothelium is the same or different from that on the smooth muscle must await the development of specific antagonists.

CYSTEINYL-LEUKOTRIENE DETECTED DURING HUMAN LUNG REPERFUSION

LTE_4 levels were not correlated with the high pulmonary arterial pressure observed in infants with PH (Figure 2). These data are similar to those obtained in a previous study in adult pulmonary hypertensive patients where other metabolites of the arachidonic acid cascade were measured[22]. These authors found no correlation between the pulmonary arterial pressure and thromboxane B_2 (TxB_2) levels in urine samples. Such data suggest that the circulating potent vasoconstrictor metabolites of the arachidonic acid pathway (TxA_2 and LTE_4) which are detected in pulmonary hypertension may not be related to the in vivo pressure modulations reported in the pulmonary artery.

The low levels of LTE_4 (undetectable in five of 18 patients) and inter-patient variation require further investigation: there may be a preferential metabolism of arachidonic acid in different individuals. A modification in the production/removal equilibrium of the 5-LO metabolites could result in alterations in detection of the more stable metabolite (LTE_4). Therefore, the measurement of only LTE_4 in the biological samples may not be an appropriate index of the 5-LO pathway activity in all patients. The considerable variation in the levels of LTE_4 between patients may also be related to the way LTE_4 is bound in the circulation. Unfortunately little is known about the fixation of cys-LTs in the human circulation. Few studies have been

***Figure 1** The cysteinyl-leukotrienes act at a single receptor (CysLT$_1$) located on the airway muscle. Stimulation of this receptor induces airway muscle contraction. This response is blocked by a variety of antagonists (CysLT$_1$-antag). In the smooth muscle of pulmonary veins another cys-LT receptor (CysLT$_2$) is present. Stimulation of this receptor produces a contraction which is not blocked by the antagonists known to be effective in airways. In addition, the endothelium contains two receptors: one (CysLT$_1$) which is associated with contraction and is blocked by the antagonists and a second receptor (CysLT$_2$) associated with relaxation via nitric oxide. This latter receptor is also resistant to the antagonists which block the airway responses*

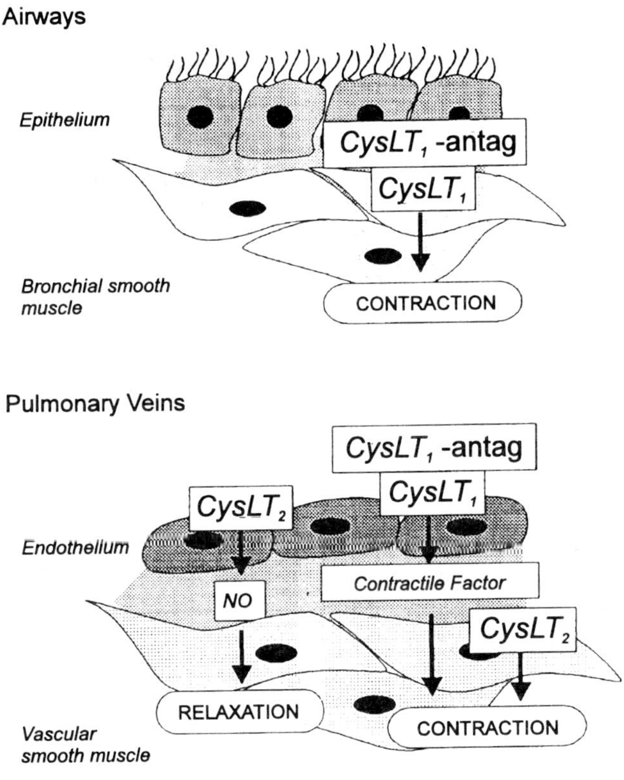

published dealing with the quantitation of cys-LTs in human blood samples and analysis has been essentially based on results derived from human plasma[23]. Finally, an increase in quantities of cys-LTs may occur in the tissue compartment rather than in the circulation. Previous data have shown that following an instillation of cys-LTs in the rat lung only a small percentage could be detected in the lavage fluid[24] suggesting that the lung tissue rather than the lung liquid was the dominant compartment. Whether or not lung tissue from pulmonary hypertensive patients exhibits elevated

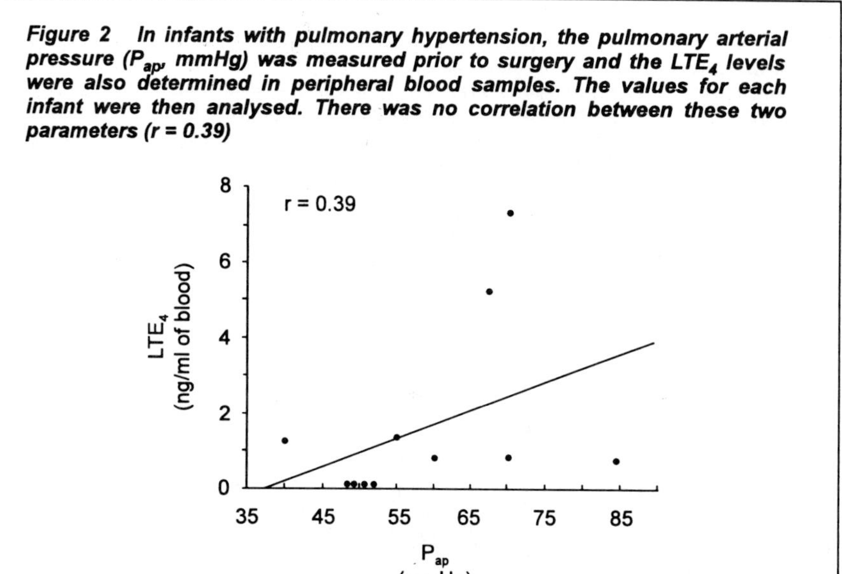

Figure 2 *In infants with pulmonary hypertension, the pulmonary arterial pressure (P_{ap}, mmHg) was measured prior to surgery and the LTE_4 levels were also determined in peripheral blood samples. The values for each infant were then analysed. There was no correlation between these two parameters (r = 0.39)*

levels of LTE_4 has not been reported. The data presented in Figure 3 suggest that there are no differences in the quantities of LTE_4 extracted from human lung tissue samples which were derived from adult patients with pulmonary hypertension.

CONCLUSIONS

An attempt has been made to determine the circulating levels of LTE_4 in infants before and during open heart surgery for correction of congenital heart lesions. The data demonstrate that this mediator can be extracted from human heparinized whole blood when collected directly into methanol. These data suggest that measurements of LTE_4 in blood samples obtained from infants may be different from that of adults. Since no increase in the circulating LTE_4 blood levels was observed in infants with PH these data suggest that the episodes of transitory pulmonary hypertension may not be associated with this metabolite. However, these measurements do not preclude the possibility of the presence of other metabolites in the transitory increases in pulmonary arterial pressure. Of some interest is the observation that the LTE_4 blood levels remained constant during the surgical intervention. These data demonstrate that mechanical manipulation and cardiac repair do not modify LTE_4 in the blood. In addition, under these conditions, the human lung in situ appears not to produce and release LTE_4 into the circulation.

Acknowledgements

Professor Claude Planché and Service de Chirurgie et Réanimation Cardiaques Pédiatriques.

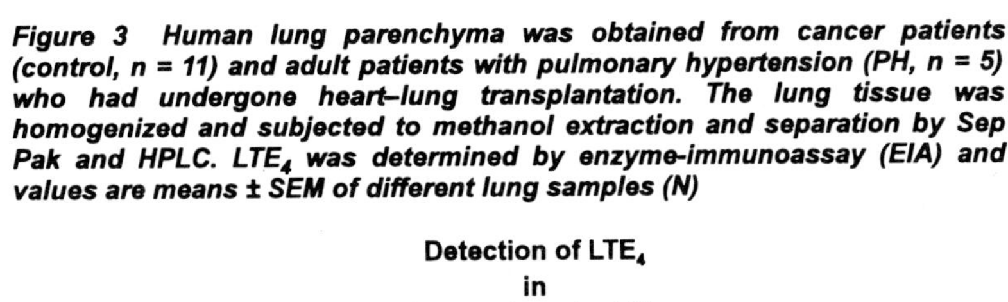

Figure 3   Human lung parenchyma was obtained from cancer patients (control, n = 11) and adult patients with pulmonary hypertension (PH, n = 5) who had undergone heart–lung transplantation. The lung tissue was homogenized and subjected to methanol extraction and separation by Sep Pak and HPLC. LTE_4 was determined by enzyme-immunoassay (EIA) and values are means ± SEM of different lung samples (N)

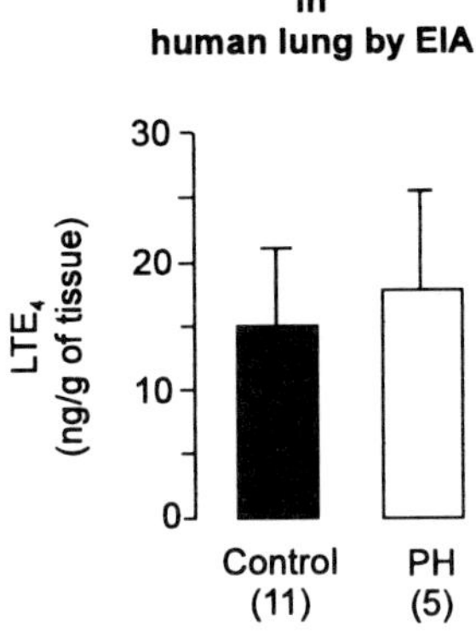

References

1. Schild HO, Hawkins DF, Mongar JL, Herxheimer H. Reactions of isolated human lung and bronchial tissue, to a specific antigen. Lancet. 1951; 261: 376–82.
2. Brocklehurst WE. The release of histamine and formation of a slow reacting substance (SRS-A) during anaphylactic shock. J Physiol. 1960; 151: 416–35.
3. Dahlén S-E, Hansson G, Hedqvist P, Bjorck T, Granstrom E, Dahlén B. Allergen challenge of lung tissue from asthmatics elicits bronchial contraction that correlates with the release of leukotrienes C4, D4 and E4. Proc Natl Acad Sci USA. 1983; 80: 1712–16.
4. Orange RP, Murphy RC, Karnovsky ML, Austen KF. The physio-chemical characteristics and purification of SRS-A. J Immunol. 1973; 110: 760–70.
5. Undem BJ, Pickett WC, Lichtenstein LM, Adams GK. The effect of indomethacin on immunologic release of histamine and sulfidopeptide leukotrienes from human bronchus and lung parenchyma. Am Rev Resp Dis. 1987; 138: 1183–7.
6. Murphy RC, Hammarström S, Samuelsson B. Leukotriene C: A slow reacting substance from murine mastocytoma cells. Proc Natl Acad Sci USA. 1979; 76: 4275–9.
7. Lam S, Chan H, Leriche JC, Chan-Yeung M, Salari H. Release of leukotrienes in patients with bronchial asthma. J Allergy Clin Immunol. 1988; 81: 711–17.
8. Taylor GW, Taylor I, Black P, et al. Urinary leukotriene E4 after antigen challenge and in acute asthma and allergic rhinitis. Lancet. 1989; 1: 584–8.
9. Sampson AP, Green CP, Spencer DA, Piper PJ, Price JF. Leukotrienes in the blood and urine of children with acute asthma. Ann NY Acad Sci. 1991; 629: 437–9.
10. Manning PJ, Rokach J, Malo JL, et al. Urinary leukotriene E_4 levels during early and late asthmatic responses. J Allergy Clin Immunol. 1990; 86: 211–20.
11. Lee TH, Crea AEG, Gant V, et al. Identification of lipoxin A_4 and its relationship to the sulfidopeptide leukotrienes C_4, D_4 and E_4 in the bronchoalveolar lavage fluids obtained from patients with selected pulmonary diseases. Am Rev Resp Dis. 1990; 141: 1453–8.
12. Stenmark KR, James SL, Voelkel NF, et al. Leukotriene C4 and D4 in neonates with hypoxemia and pulmonary hypertension. N Engl J Med. 1983; 309: 77–80.

13. Serraf A, Bruniaux J, Lacourt-Gayet F, et al. Obstructed total anomalous pulmonary venous return. J Thorac Cardiovasc Surg. 1991; 101: 601–6.
14. Berkowitz BA, Zabko-Potapovich B, Volocik R, Gleason JG. Effects of the leukotrienes on the vasculature and blood pressure of different species. J Pharmacol Exp Ther. 1984; 229: 105–12.
15. Gause GE, Baker R, Cassin S. Specificity of FPL 57231 for leukotriene receptors in fetal pulmonary circulation. Am J Physiol. 1988; 254: 120–5.
16. Secrest RJ, Ohlstein EH, Chapnick BM. Leukotriene D4 relaxes canine renal and superior mesenteric arteries. Circ Res. 1985; 57: 323–9.
17. Secrest RJ, Ohlstein EH, Chapnick BM. Relationship between LTD4-induced endothelium-dependent vasomotor relaxation and cGMP. J Pharmacol Exp Ther. 1988; 245: 47–52.
18. Sakuma I, Levi R. Vasomotor effects of leukotriene C4 and D4 on cavian pulmonary artery and aorta. Ann NY Acad Sci. 1988; 524: 91–102.
19. Ortiz JL, Gorenne I, Cortijo J, et al. Leukotriene receptors on human pulmonary vascular endothelium. Br J Pharmacol. 1995; 115: 1382–6.
20. Gorenne I, Norel X, Brink C. Cysteinyl-leukotriene receptors in the human lung: what's new? TiPS. 1996; 17: 342–5.
21. Labat C, Ortiz JL, Norel X, et al. A second cysteinyl leukotriene receptor in human lung. J Pharmacol Exp Ther. 1992; 63: 800–5
22. Christman BW, McPherson CD, Newman JH et al. An imbalance between the excretion of thromboxane and prostacyclin metabolites in pulmonary hypertension. N Engl J Med. 1992; 327: 70–5.
23. Heavey DJ, Soberman RJ, Lewis RA, Spur B, Austen KF. Critical considerations in the development of an assay for sulfidopeptide leukotrienes in plasma. Prostaglandins. 1987; 33: 693–705.
24. Wescolt JY, McDonnell TJ, Voekel NF. Alveolar transfer and metabolism of eicosanoids in the rat. Am Rev Resp Dis. 1989; 139: 80–7.

13 Leukotrienes in cardiovascular disease

A. SALA

Cysteinyl-leukotrienes (cys-LTs, LTC_4, LTD_4 and LTE_4) are potent lipid mediators, resulting from the oxidative metabolism of arachidonic acid through the 5-lipoxygenase (5-LO) pathway. They are able to affect all major components of the cardiovascular system: they can constrict small and large vessels, modify cardiac and coronary functions, influence the microcirculation and contribute to the manifestations of ischaemia/reperfusion injury[1,2]. Furthermore cys-LTs are able to induce profound modification of vascular permeability, leading to oedema formation[3].

Cys-LT biosynthesis is dependent on the activity of the 5-LO enzyme, a single protein possessing the dioxygenase activity necessary for the synthesis of 5-hydroperoxy eicosatetraenoic acid (5-HpETE), and the epoxygenase activity leading to leukotriene A_4 (LTA_4)[4]. This unstable allylic epoxide can be further converted by two different enzymes: LTA_4 hydrolase, catalysing the conversion into leukotriene B_4 (LTB_4), and leukotriene C_4 synthase, responsible for the specific introduction of a molecule of glutathione on LTA_4 resulting in the formation of leukotriene C_4 (LTC_4)[5]. The distribution of these secondary enzymes characterizes the final product of 5-LO activation in different cellular species: neutrophils generate predominantly LTB_4, a compound with very potent chemo-attractant activities[6], while eosinophils and mast-cells[7,8] show preferential production of cys-LT. Recently it has been shown that the secondary enzymes (i.e. LTA_4 hydrolase and LTC_4 synthase) are also expressed by cells which do not contain the primary oxidative enzyme, (5-LO). Erythrocytes, platelets, and endothelial cells (EC) are indeed able to take up the unstable metabolic intermediate LTA_4 and convert it into LTB_4 (erythrocytes) or LTC_4 (EC and platelets) It has been known for many years that neutrophils and mast cells, which possess a very active 5-LO, release extracellularly substantial amounts of unmetabolized LTA_4. Taken together these observations led to experiments proving the cooperation of different cells for the biosynthesis of biologically active leukotrienes [9–13]. This type of biosynthetic reaction involving the cooperation of different cell types has been named transcellular synthesis, and it supports the hypothesis that the cellular environment (cell–cell interactions) may affect both quantitatively and qualitatively the profile of metabolites resulting from the activation of 5-LO-bearing cells[14].

TRANSCELLULAR SYNTHESIS OF cys-LT IN ISOLATED, POLYMORPHONUCLEAR LEUCOCYTE-PERFUSED RABBIT HEART

We have developed a model of spontaneously beating, isolated rabbit heart, perfused with purified human polymorphonuclear leukocytes (PMNL) showing that PMNL activation causes cys-LT formation through PMNL-EC transcellular synthesis, resulting in increased coronary resistance and cardiac damage[15,16]. Rabbit heart-Langendorff preparations at constant flow, perfused with purified human PMNL and challenged with the calcium ionophore A23187 (0.5 μM, 30 minutes), produce substantial amounts of cys-LTs[15]. Similar results are obtained perfusing PMNL primed with granulocyte-macrophage colony stimulating factor (GM-CSF, 1 nM, 30 minutes) and challenged with the formylated tripeptide fMLP (1 μM, 60 minutes)[16]. Comparison of 5-LO metabolites observed in PMNL-perfused rabbit hearts with that synthesized upon challenge of isolated PMNL shows decreased amounts of LTB_4 and its ω-oxidized metabolites in heart perfusates; this is accompanied by a several-fold increase in cys-LTs, in spite of negligible production of cys-LTs by the heart alone. Inhibition of PMNL 5-LO only, using the slowly reversible LT biosynthesis inhibitor compound MK-886[17] followed by washing of the PMNL before perfusion through the isolated heart, resulted in levels of cys-LTs in the recirculating medium barely distinguishable from that contributed by the heart alone. This indicates that the amounts of cys-LTs detected upon addition of untreated PMNL to the isolated heart are the result of PMNL 5-LO activation, in spite of the fact that the cys-LTs cannot be contributed by the PMNL themselves[15]. Taken together these data strongly support the hypothesis of a cooperation of PMNL with the coronary EC for the production of significant amounts of cys-LT involving the transfer of LTA_4 from PMNL to EC.

The observed shift from LTA_4-hydrolase metabolites to cys-LT moving from isolated PMNL to PMNL perfusing the isolated heart preparation, suggests that relevant amounts of LTB_4 and ω-oxidized LTB_4 metabolites observed upon challenge in isolated cell preparations are the result of the release of LTA_4 and further metabolism to LTB_4 by surrounding PMNL. In agreement with this hypothesis we showed that intact LTB_4 indeed represents the main LTA_4-metabolite released by human PMNL upon challenge with the Ca-ionophore A23187[18].

EFFECT OF TRANSCELLULAR SYNTHESIS OF cys-LT ON CARDIAC FUNCTION AND MORPHOLOGY

Activation of PMNL in perfused rabbit hearts induces progressive increase of coronary perfusion pressure (CPP; 150–300% over basal values, 30 minutes after challenge), as well as left-ventricular end-diastolic pressure (LVEDP; 200–700% over basal values), suggesting the onset of coronary vasospasm and decreased microvascular patency. The hypothesis of a causal relationship between production of cys-LTs and coronary vasoconstriction is in agreement with the known vasoconstricting action of cys-LTs[1,2,19] and is supported by the effect of two different cys-LT receptor antagonists LY171883 (10 μM)[20] and SKF104353 (10 μM)[21], which are able to inhibit significantly the changes in CPP following PMNL activation.

In agreement with the potent effect of cys-LTs on microvascular permeability[3], morphological analysis by light and electron microscopy of PMNL-perfused rabbit hearts shows the presence of activated EC and perivascular oedema. Morphological changes are also prevented by pretreatment with the LTD_4 receptor antagonist

SKF104353 as well as by the LT biosynthesis inhibitor MK-886, further supporting the cardinal role of cys-LTs in the overall cardiac derangement observed upon PMNL activation.

CELL–CELL INTERACTION, cys-LT SYNTHESIS AND CARDIOVASCULAR INFLAMMATION

It has been recognized for many years that the adhesion of PMNL to microvascular endothelium is a crucial event in inflammatory reactions and in cardiovascular diseases: cell–cell interactions mediated by intercellular adhesion molecules[22,23] are likely to play an active role for the anchoring of circulating cells that characterizes the beginning of the cellular contribution to inflammatory reactions. Adhesion of neutrophils to endothelial cells may also represent an optimal condition for transcellular biosynthesis of cys-LT, leading to a very efficient transfer of LTA_4 from one cell to the other. Recently, Brady and Serhan reported on the transcellular synthesis of cys-LTs in PMNL-glomerular EC co-incubations[24]. In this model, cys-LT formation was significantly blunted in the presence of monoclonal antibodies directed against CD11/CD18 integrins and L-selectin, providing the grounds for the hypothesis that adhesion molecule-mediated cell–cell interactions facilitate cys-LT biosynthesis: adhering membranes may represent a lipophilic environment allowing the transfer of intact LTA_4 from PMNL to EC. Support for this hypothesis is also provided by the observed stabilization of intact LTA_4 by membrane-like liposomes[25].

Nitric oxide (NO), formerly known as endothelium derived-relaxing factor[26], is a labile compound inducing increased level of intracellular cGMP in various tissues that causes vascular smooth muscle relaxation, and profound hypotension in anaesthetized animals (reviewed in 27). Furthermore, NO is able to inhibit platelet aggregation, reduce platelet adhesion to endothelial cells in vitro and inhibit PMN aggregation[28,29].

An increasing amount of evidence pointed to a possible role of NO as an endogenous modulator of leukocyte adhesion[30] (reviewed in 31). Pretreatment of the isolated rabbit heart with the NO synthase inhibitor L-NMMA[32], at a dose resulting in 100% increase of the basal CPP (10 µM), followed by perfusion of PMNL and challenge, caused a very rapid adhesion of PMNL associated with synthesis of large amounts of cys-LT and a dramatic increase in CPP (Figure 1). Restoration of NO synthesis with L-arginine pretreatment (100 µM), significantly decreased the challenge-induced adhesion of perfusing PMNL. This effect resulted in a significant reduction of cys-LT production as well as in the associated changes in CPP, supporting the importance of PMNL-EC adhesion toward transcellular synthesis of cys-LTs (Figure 2)[33].

CONCLUSIONS

Evidence for cys-LT transcellular synthesis by PMNL-EC cooperation has been documented using isolated cell preparations[11,24], as well as in a more complex model of pulmonary leukostasis in the isolated, perfused rabbit lung[34], but it has never been

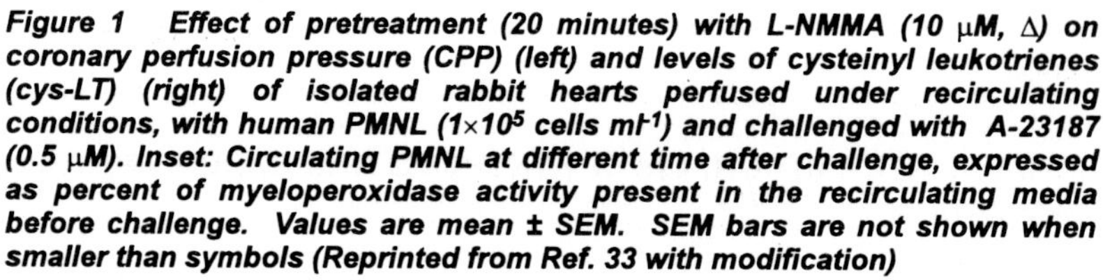

Figure 1   Effect of pretreatment (20 minutes) with L-NMMA (10 µM, Δ) on coronary perfusion pressure (CPP) (left) and levels of cysteinyl leukotrienes (cys-LT) (right) of isolated rabbit hearts perfused under recirculating conditions, with human PMNL (1×10⁵ cells ml⁻¹) and challenged with A-23187 (0.5 µM). Inset: Circulating PMNL at different time after challenge, expressed as percent of myeloperoxidase activity present in the recirculating media before challenge. Values are mean ± SEM. SEM bars are not shown when smaller than symbols (Reprinted from Ref. 33 with modification)

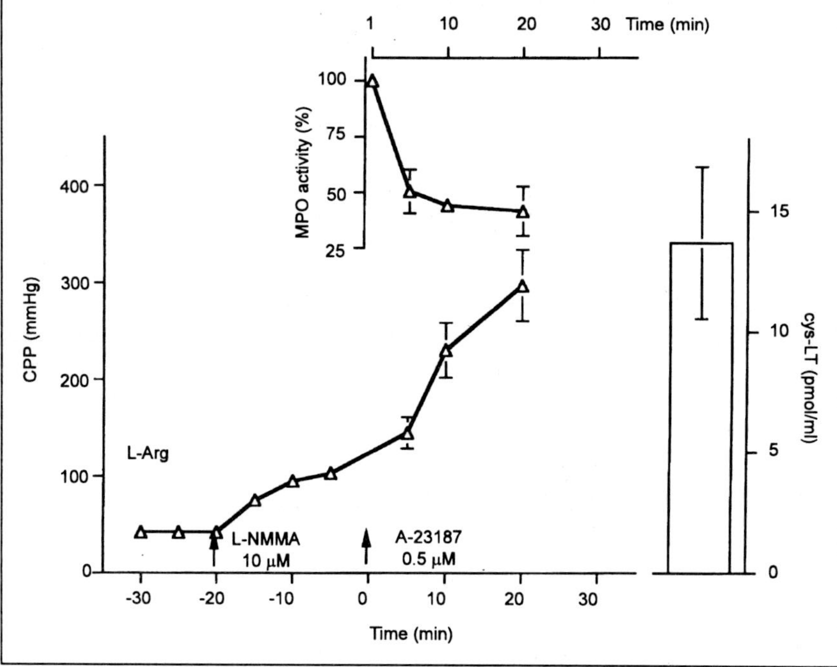

addressed for cardiovascular functions. Local formation of cys-LTs via transcellular synthesis causes important functional changes and morphological modifications in a model of PMNL-perfused isolated rabbit heart. The conversion of LTA_4 into cys-LTs at the level of the vessel walls may result in elevated local concentrations of mediators at effector sites, e.g. smooth muscle cells adjacent to the EC lining.

The experimental evidence obtained confirms the role of NO as a potential endogenous modulator of PMNL-EC adhesion and provides unequivocal evidence for the importance of cell–cell adhesion towards the transfer of intact LTA_4 required for transcellular synthesis of cys-LTs. Therefore the complex interplay between promoters (thrombin, TNF)[35,36] and inhibitors (PGI$_2$, NO)[37] of leukocyte adhesion, may ultimately result in different biosynthetic profiles of metabolism of arachidonic acid. It is important to note that the cys-LTs resulting from PMNL-EC transcellular synthesis are able to amplify their own production, inducing EC dependent neutrophil adhesion[38] and subsequent additional transcellular synthesis of cys-LTs.

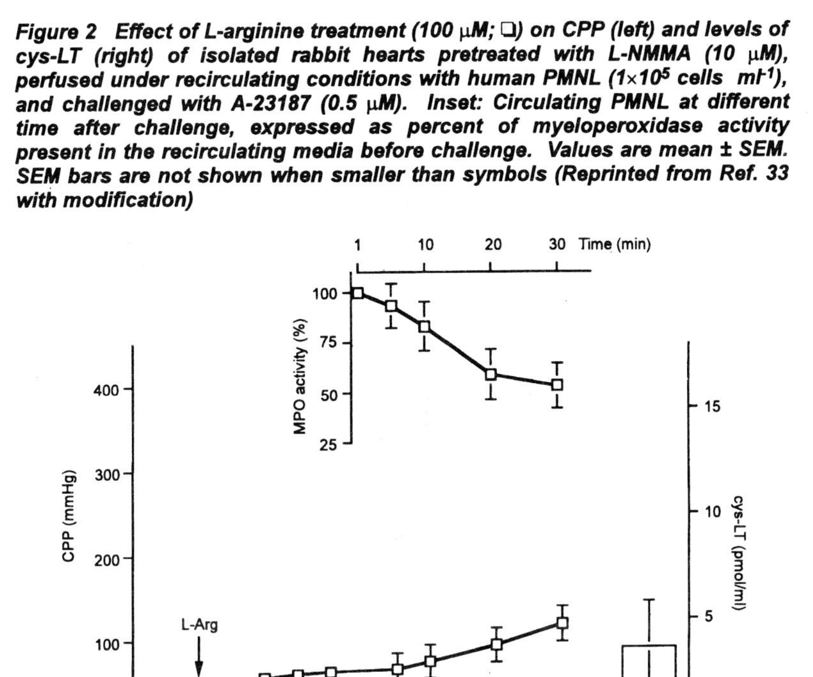

Figure 2 *Effect of L-arginine treatment (100 μM; □) on CPP (left) and levels of cys-LT (right) of isolated rabbit hearts pretreated with L-NMMA (10 μM), perfused under recirculating conditions with human PMNL (1×10⁵ cells ml⁻¹), and challenged with A-23187 (0.5 μM). Inset: Circulating PMNL at different time after challenge, expressed as percent of myeloperoxidase activity present in the recirculating media before challenge. Values are mean ± SEM. SEM bars are not shown when smaller than symbols (Reprinted from Ref. 33 with modification)*

The mechanisms described add a novel aspect to the potential role of PMNL in ischaemic vascular disease (reviewed in 39), and provide the grounds for a reassessment of neutrophil-derived mediators in ischaemia-reperfusion injury[40,41]. Adhesion and activation of PMNL by hypoxic human EC[42] may represent the trigger for the transcellular synthesis of relevant amounts of cys-LTs within reperfused areas, leading to the hypothesis of a significant contribution of cys-LTs to PMNL-dependent vascular damage. Furthermore, the increase in permeability and the expression of cell-surface adhesive glycoproteins such as ICAM-1 are among the changes observed in the endothelium during the early phases of atherogenesis[43,44]. These observations may find a common link in the transcellular synthesis of cys-LTs by adhering leukocyte-EC cooperation. Modulation of PMNL adhesion may thus represent a novel approach to the pharmacological control of the biosynthesis of cys-LTs.

Acknowledgements

The work presented here constitutes the combined effort of researchers from the Center for Cardiopulmonary Pharmacology, including Giuseppe Rossoni, Carola

Buccellati, Albino Bonazzi, Ferruccio Berti and Giancarlo Folco. Supported in part by the EEC grant CT93 1533.

References

1. Roth DM, Lefer AM. Studies on the mechanism of leukotriene induced coronary artery constriction. Prostaglandins. 1983;26:573–81.
2. Piper PJ, Samhoun MN. Leukotrienes. Br Med Bull. 1987;43:297–311.
3. Dahlén S-E, Bjork J, Hedquist P, et al. Leukotrienes promote plasma leakage and leukocyte adhesion in post-capillary venules: In vivo effects with relevance to the acute inflammatory response. Proc Natl Acad Sci USA. 1981;78:3887–91.
4. Shimizu T, Rådmark O, Samuelsson B. Enzyme with dual lipoxygenase activities catalyzes leukotriene A4 synthesis from arachidonic acid. Proc Natl Acad Sci USA. 1984;81:689–93.
5. Lewis RA, Austen KF. The biologically active leukotrienes: Biosynthesis, metabolism, receptors, functions and pharmacology. J Clin Invest. 1984;73:889–97.
6. Borgeat P, Samuelsson B. Arachidonic acid metabolism in polymorphonuclear leukocytes: Effects of ionophore A23187. Proc Natl Acad Sci USA. 1979;76:2148–52.
7. Weller PF, Lee CW, Foster DW, Corey EJ, Austen KF, Lewis RA. Generation and metabolism of 5-lipoxygenase pathway leukotrienes by human eosinophils: Predominant production of leukotriene C_4. Proc Natl Acad Sci USA. 1983;80:7626–30.
8. MacGlashan DW Jr, Schleimer RP, Peters SP, Schulman ES, Adams GK 3rd, Newball HH, Lichtenstein LM. Generation of leukotrienes by purified human lung mast cells. J Clin Invest. 1982;70:747–51.
9. McGee JE, Fitzpatrick FA. Erythrocyte-neutrophil interaction: Formation of leukotriene B_4 by transcellular biosynthesis. Proc Natl Acad Sci USA. 1986;83:1349–53.
10. Maclouf JA, Murphy RC. Transcellular metabolism of neutrophil-derived leukotriene A_4 by human platelets. J Biol Chem. 1988,263:174–81.
11. Feinmark SJ, Cannon PJ. Endothelial cell leukotriene C_4 synthesis results from intracellular transfer of leukotriene A_4 synthesized by polymorphonuclear leukocytes. J Biol Chem. 1986;261:16466–72.
12. Claesson HE, Haeggström J. Human endothelial cells stimulate leukotriene synthesis and convert granulocyte-released leukotriene A_4 into leukotrienes B_4, C_4, D_4 and E_4. Eur J Biochem. 1988;173:93–100.
13. Marcus AJ, Broekman MJ, Safier LB, et al. Formation of leukotriene and other hydroxyacids during platelet-neutrophil interactions in vitro. Biochem Biophys Res Commun. 1982;109:30–8.
14. Maclouf J, Murphy RC, Henson P. Transcellular sulfidopeptide leukotriene biosynthetic capacity of vascular cells. Blood. 1989;74:703–7.
15. Sala A, Rossoni G, Buccellati C, Berti F, Maclouf J, Folco GC. Formation of sulfidopeptide-leukotrienes by cell–cell interaction causes coronary vasoconstriction in isolated, cell-perfused rabbit heart. Br J Pharmacol. 1993;110:1206–12.
16. Sala A, Aliev GM, Rossoni G, et al. Morphological and functional changes of coronary vasculature caused by transcellular biosynthesis of sulfidopeptide leukotrienes in isolated heart of rabbit. Blood. 1996;87:1824–32.
17. Gillard J, Ford-Hutchinson AW, Chan C, et al. L-663, 536 (MK-886) (3-(1-(4-chlorobenzyl)-3-*t*-butyl-thio-5-isopropylindol-2-yl)-2,2-dimethylpropanoic acid), a novel orally active leukotriene biosynthesis inhibitor. Can J Physiol Pharmacol. 1989;67:456–64.
18. Sala A, Bolla M, Zarini S, Müller-Peddinghaus R, Folco G. Release of leukotriene A_4 versus leukotriene B_4 from human polymorphonuclear leukocytes. J Biol Chem. 1996;271;17944–8.
19. Michelassi F, Landa L, Hill RD, et al. Leukotriene D_4: A potent coronary artery vasoconstrictor associated with impaired ventricular contraction. Science. 1982;217:841–3.
20. Fleish JH, Rinkema LE, Haisch KD, et al. LY171883,1-(2-hydroxy-3-propyl-4-(4-(1H-tetrazol-5yl)butoxy)phenyl)ethanone, an orally active leukotriene D_4 antagonist. J Pharmacol Exp Ther. 1985;233:148–57.
21. Mong S, Wu HL, Miller J, Hall RF, Gleason JG, Crooke ST. SKF104353, a high affinity

antagonist for human and guinea-pig lung LTD_4 receptor, blocked phosphatidylinositol metabolism and thromboxane synthesis induced by leukotriene D_4. Mol Pharmacol. 1987;32,223–9.

22. Hynes RO. Integrins: Versatility, modulation, and signalling in cell adhesion. Cell. 1992;69:11–25.

23. Makgoba MW, Bernard A, Sanders ME. Cell adhesion/signalling: Biology and clinical applications. Eur J Clin Invest. 1992;22:443–53.

24. Brady HR, Serhan CN. Adhesion promotes transcellular leukotriene biosynthesis during neutrophil-glomerular endothelial cell interactions: Inhibition by antibodies against CD18 and L-selectin. Biochem Biophys Res Commun. 1992;186:1307–14.

25. Fiore S, Serhan CN. Phospholipid bilayers enhance the stability of leukotriene A_4 and epoxytetraenes: Stabilization of eicosanoids by liposomes. Biochem Biophys Res Commun. 1989;159:477–81.

26. Palmer RM, Ferrige AG, Moncada S. Nitric oxide release accounts for the biological activity of endothelium-derived relaxing factor. Nature. 1987;327:524–6.

27. Moncada S. Nitric oxide. J Hypertension. 1994;12:S359.

28. Radomski MW, Palmer RM, Moncada S. Endogenous nitric oxide inhibits human platelet adhesion to vascular endothelium. Lancet. 1987;2:1057–8.

29. Radomski MW, Palmer RM, Moncada S. Comparative pharmacology of endothelium-derived relaxing factor, nitric oxide and prostacyclin in platelets. Br J Pharmacol. 1987;92:181–7.

30. Kubes P, Suzuki M, Granger DN. Nitric oxide: An endogenous modulator of leukocyte adhesion. Proc Natl Acad Sci USA. 1991;88:4651–5.

31. Lefer AM, Lefer DJ. The role of nitric oxide and cell adhesion molecules on the microcirculation in ischaemia-reperfusion. Cardiovasc Res. 1996;32:743–51.

32. Palmer RM, Moncada S. A novel citrulline-forming enzyme implicated in the formation of nitric oxide by vascular endothelial cells. Biochem Biophys Res Commun. 1989;158:348–52.

33. Buccellati C, Rossoni G, Bonazzi A, et al. Nitric oxide modulates transcellular biosynthesis of cys-leukotrienes in leukocyte-perfused rabbit heart. Br J Pharmacol. 1997;120:1128–34.

34. Grimminger F, Kreusler B, Schneider U, Becker G, Seeger W. Influence of microvascular adherence on neutrophil leukotriene generation. J Immunol. 1990;144:1866–72.

35. Lo SK, Everitt J, Gu J, Malik AB. Tumor necrosis factor mediates experimental pulmonary edema by ICAM-1 and CD18-dependent mechanisms. J Clin Invest. 1992;89:981–8.

36. Sugama Y, Tiruppati C, Janakidevi K, Andersen TT, Fenton JW, Malik AB. Thrombin-induced expression of endothelial P-selectin and intercellular adhesion molecule-1: A mechanism for stabilizing neutrophil adhesion. J Cell Biol. 1992;119:935–44.

37. Erlansson M, Bergqvist D, Persson NH, Svensjo E. Modification of postischemic increase of leukocyte adhesion and vascular permeability in the hamster by iloprost. Prostaglandins. 1991;41:157–68.

38. Zimmerman GA, Prescott SM, McIntyre TM. Leukotrienes C_4 and D_4 stimulate human endothelial cells to synthesize platelet-activating factor and bind neutrophils. Proc Natl Acad Sci USA. 1986;83:2204–8.

39. Hansen PR. Role of neutrophils in myocardial ischemia and reperfusion. Circulation. 1995;91:1872–85.

40. Evers AS, Murphree S, Saffitz JE, Jakschik BA, Needleman, P. Effects of endogenously produced leukotrienes, thromboxane and prostaglandins on coronary vascular resistance in rabbit myocardial infarction. J Clin Invest. 1985;75:992–9.

41. Mullane K. Myocardial ischemia-reperfusion injury: role of neutrophils and neutrophil derived mediators. In: Marone G, Lichtenstein LM, Condorelli M, Fauci AS, editors. Human Inflammatory Disease – Clinical Immunology. Toronto: BC Deckers, 1988:143–60.

42. Arnould T, Michiels C, Remacle J. Hypoxic human umbilical vein endothelial cells induce activation of adherent polymorphonuclear leukocytes. Blood. 1994;83:3705–16.

43. Simionescu N, Vasile E, Lupu F, Popescu G, Simionescu M. Prelesional events in atherogenesis. Accumulation of extracellular cholesterol-rich liposomes in the arterial intima and cardiac valves of the hyperlipidemic rabbit. Am J Pathol. 1986;123:109–25.

44. Sawamura T, Kume N, Aoyama T, et al. An endothelial receptor for oxidized low-density lipoprotein. Nature. 1997;385:73–7.

14 Leukotriene B$_4$: agonist for the fat regulator PPARα

P.R. DEVCHAND and W. WAHLI

Control of an inflammatory response is primarily achieved by 'turning off' or inactivating the signals that help to recruit cells of the immune system to the site of inflammation. Many inflammatory disorders underscore the importance of turnover of signals including the broad set of arachidonic acid metabolites. One such fatty acid derivative, leukotriene B$_4$(LTB$_4$) is a potent chemotactic agent whose activity is mediated by a membrane receptor[1]. Two approaches can be used to gain therapeutic or exogenous control over LTB$_4$-mediated inflammation. The first, is to inhibit the LTB$_4$ signal by administration of drugs that act either as LTB$_4$ membrane receptor antagonists or biosynthesis inhibitors. Indeed, this is a valid approach and many banks of synthetic LTB$_4$ membrane receptor antagonists and biosynthesis inhibitors have been established. The second approach is to reduce the level of LTB$_4$ by increasing its metabolism. In vitro, two types of compounds have been shown to modulate LTB$_4$ metabolism: dietary ω-3 polyunsaturated fatty acids[2] and the lipid lowering drug, clofibrate[3]. The mechanism(s) by which these compounds lower the levels of LTB$_4$ to exert an anti-inflammatory effect have until recently, been elusive.

CATABOLISM OF LTB$_4$ BY FATTY ACID OXIDATION PATHWAYS

Inactivation of LTB$_4$ can be achieved simply by its catabolism via the fatty acid ω- and β-oxidation pathways, in microsomes and peroxisomes respectively[4] These pathways are capable of handling a broad spectrum of substrates, ranging from lipid lowering drugs to fatty acids and their derivatives (Figure 1). In response to an overload of substrate, enzymes of these oxidation pathways are up-regulated at the transcriptional level (for review see 5). When challenged with high doses of substrate, rodents often respond by proliferation of peroxisomes in the liver. Compounds that induce this response are termed peroxisome proliferators.

FROM DRUG DETOXIFIER TO FAT CONTROLLER

In a screen for the factors that mediate peroxisome proliferation a cDNA coding for the mouse peroxisome proliferator-activated receptor (PPAR) was isolated[6]. Sequence analyses revealed that PPAR is a transcription factor that belongs to the nuclear hormone receptor (NHR) superfamily. By analogy to NHRs, the PPAR protein can be depicted as an assembly of functional regions for DNA binding, ligand binding

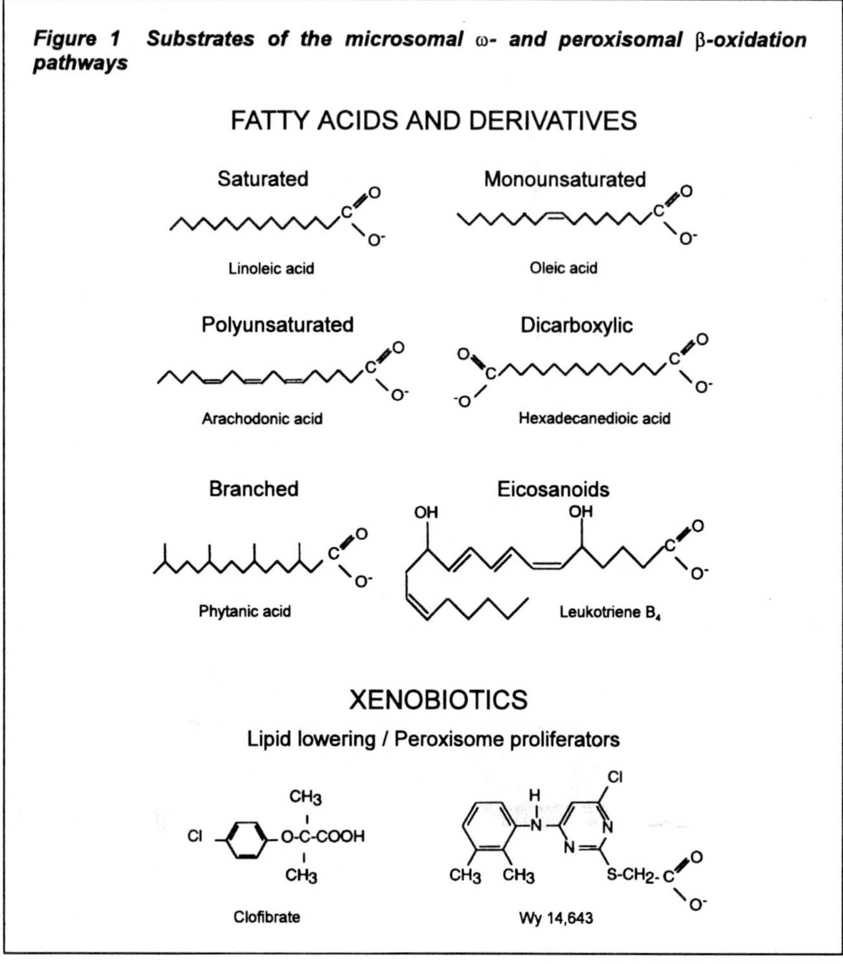

and transcriptional activation. The isolation and characterization of three related PPAR cDNAs (α, β and γ) from *Xenopus* revealed that PPARs represent a distinct subfamily of NHRs[7].

PPARs regulate transcription as a heterodimeric complex with another NHR, the 9-*cis* retinoic acid receptor (RXR). The PPAR-RXR heterodimer recognises defined short DNA sequences (peroxisome proliferator response elements or PPREs) in the promoter of target genes. This regulatory system is ligand-inducible, that is, transcription of target genes is up-regulated in response to a signal which binds directly to the receptor (Figure 2). The target genes of PPARs are involved in many aspects of lipid biology such as fatty acid trafficking, storage and metabolism. Hence the prediction that PPARs play a key role in maintaining lipid and energy homoeostasis (for comprehensive reviews see 8–10).

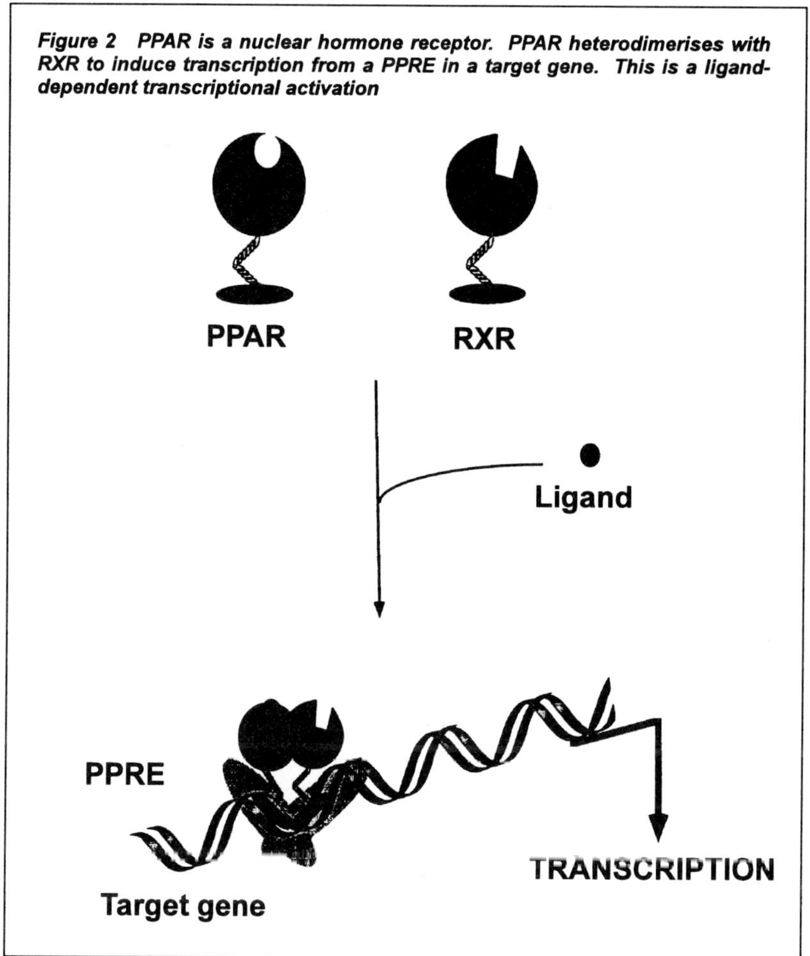

Figure 2 *PPAR is a nuclear hormone receptor. PPAR heterodimerises with RXR to induce transcription from a PPRE in a target gene. This is a ligand-dependent transcriptional activation*

PPARα ACTIVATORS

A standard assay for evaluating the effect of a compound on PPAR activity is the transient transfection assay. Cells are transfected with three constructs: an expression plasmid for PPAR, a reporter plasmid containing a PPRE-driven gene that can be easily evaluated, for example chloramphenicol acetyl transferase (CAT), and an internal standard to normalize between different samples. The cells are then exposed to a test compound for 24–48 h, harvested and evaluated. A compound which results in an increased activity of the CAT reporter is termed an activator.

Transient transfection assays have proved to be an efficient way to screen for PPAR activators (see 10 for review). Amongst the activators of PPARα are lipid lowering drugs of the fibrate class, polyunsaturated fatty acids (PUFAs) and eicosanoid signalling molecules including LTB₄, carba-prostacyclin and 8S-HETE[10].

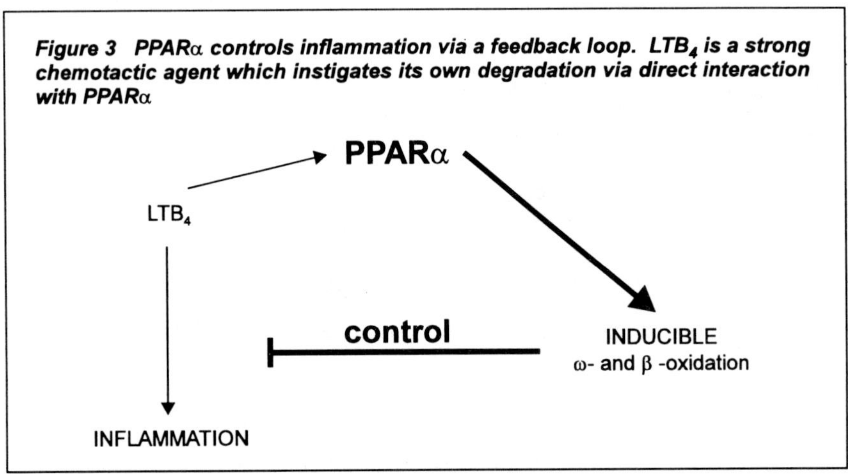

Figure 3   PPARα controls inflammation via a feedback loop. LTB₄ is a strong chemotactic agent which instigates its own degradation via direct interaction with PPARα

PPARα LIGANDS

A positive test compound could potentially activate PPAR either directly, by binding to the nuclear receptor as a ligand and/or indirectly by one of many avenues, for example, production of a metabolite which acts as a PPAR ligand. The transient transfection assays cannot distinguish between the direct and indirect mechanisms of activation.

Of the many activators, the first ligands reported for PPARα were LTB$_4$ and the lipid-lowering drug Wy 14,643[11]. We now have a large repertoire of ligands that were identified by different methods ranging from radiolabelled binding assays to semi-functional ligand-dependent assays[12–15]. One example of a semi-functional assay is the co-activator dependent receptor ligand assay (CARLA). CARLA takes advantage of a system where interaction between PPAR and the co-activator SRC-1 occurs only in the presence of ligand. This assay allows not only the affirmation of whether a compound is a ligand, but also provides a qualitative measure of ligand-PPAR affinity[15]. The PPARα ligands identified to date, encompass structurally diverse compounds including fibrates, PUFAs and eicosanoids.

PPARα AND DETOXIFICATION IN THE LIVER

The generation of a PPARα knock-out mouse has certainly accelerated evaluation of this PPAR subtype[16]. Despite the fact that these mice lack PPARα protein, under laboratory conditions they develop and reproduce normally. Further analyses indicate that when challenged with xenobiotics, the PPARα (–/–) mice are unable to increase transcription of the normal array of target genes, such as those of the microsomal ω- and peroxisomal β-oxidation pathways. These mice also do not display the normal response of peroxisomal proliferation in the liver.

The liver is an important site for clearance of natural fatty acid derived signalling molecules from the blood. RNase protection experiments in primary hepatocytes

Figure 4 *PPARα is a promising target for therapy. PPARα can be modulated by a variety of factors. It controls transcription of a battery of genes involved in inflammation control, lipid homoeostasis and liver detoxification. Hence, the model that PPARα is a good candidate for a target in the treatment of disorders associated with these functions. (CVD, cardiovascular disease)*

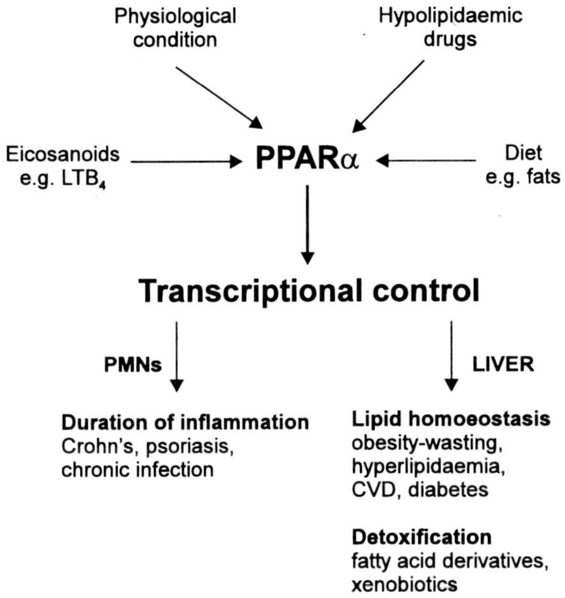

Physiological condition

Hypolipidaemic drugs

Eicosanoids e.g. LTB₄ ⟶ **PPARα** ⟵ Diet e.g. fats

Transcriptional control

PMNs

LIVER

Duration of inflammation
Crohn's, psoriasis, chronic infection

Lipid homoeostasis
obesity-wasting, hyperlipidaemia, CVD, diabetes

Detoxification
fatty acid derivatives, xenobiotics

indicate that in this biological context, LTB₄ induces transcription of acyl co-A oxidase, the well-characterized PPARα target gene and also the rate limiting enzyme of the peroxisomal β-oxidation pathway[11].

PPARα AND INFLAMMATION CONTROL

The turnover of LTB₄ is most relevant at the site of inflammation. The mouse ear swelling test reveals that compared to wild-type mice, the PPARα (–/–) knock-out mice are less efficient at clearing an arachidonic acid- or LTB₄- mediated inflammatory response[11]

Taken together with results of in vitro studies which indicate that LTB₄ binds and activates PPARα, the hepatocyte and inflammation assays suggest that LTB₄ controls its own degradation via a feedback loop: LTB₄ binds to PPARα to induce expression of enzymes of the ω- and β-oxidation pathways, ultimately resulting in increased catabolism of LTB₄ (Figure 3). In the PPARα (–/–) mouse where the transcriptional regulator is absent, the catabolic pathways are not induced, hence the inflammation is prolonged.

PPARα TARGET FOR THERAPY

PPARα is a transcription factor that senses key factors in our environment: stress, diurnal rhythm, diet and xenobiotics such as lipid lowering drugs. In response, it acts at the transcriptional level as a master director of processes that will ultimately restore homoeostasis. With a combination of diet control, drug design and tissue targeting, there are three broad areas in which PPARα shows promise in therapy: inflammation control, lipid homoeostasis and detoxification of xenobiotics or naturally occurring signalling eicosanoids (Figure 4). The ability of PPARα to recognize and react to such a broad range of structures provides ample flexibility in the development of safe drugs for prominent metabolic disorders.

References

1. Yokomizo T, Izumi T, Chang K, Takuwa Y, Shimizu T. A G-protein-coupled receptor for leukotriene B_4 that mediates chemotaxis. Nature. 1997;387:620–4.
2. von Schacky C, Kiefl R, Marcus AJ, Breokman MJ, Kaminski WE. Dietary n-3 fatty acids accelerate catabolism of leukotriene B_4 in human granulocytes. Biochim Biophys Acta. 1993;1166:20–4.
3. Couve AO, Koenig C, Santos MJ. Induction of peroxisomal enzymes and a 64-kDa peptide in cultured mouse macrophages treated with clofibrate. Exp Cell Res. 1992;202:541–4.
4. Jedlitschky G, Mayatepek E, Keppler D. Peroxisomal leukotriene degradation: Biochemical and clinical implications. Adv Enzyme Reg. 1993;33:181–94.
5. Desvergne B, Wahli W. In: Bæuerle, P, editor. Inducible transcription. Boston: Birkhäuser;1995:142–76.
6. Issemann I, Green S. Activation of a member of the steroid hormone receptor superfamily by peroxisome proliferators. Nature. 1990;347:645–50.
7. Dreyer C, Krey G, Keller H, Givel F, Helftenbein G, Wahli W. Control of the peroxisomal β-oxidation pathway by a novel family of nuclear hormone receptors. Cell. 1992;68:879–87.
8. Lemberger T, Desvergne B, Wahli W. Peroxisome proliferator-activated receptors: A nuclear receptor signaling pathway in lipid physiology. Annu Rev Cell Dev Biol. 1996;12:335–63.
9. Spiegelman BM, Flier JS. Adipogenesis and obesity: Rounding out the big picture. Cell. 1996;87:377–89.
10. Devchand PR, Wahli W. PPARα: Tempting fate with fat. In O'Malley B, editor. Hormones and Signalling. San Diego: Academic Press; 1997:235–56.
11. Devchand PR, Keller H, Peters JM, Vazquez M, Gonzalez FJ, Wahli W. The PPARalpha-leukotriene B4 pathway to inflammation control. Nature. 1996;384:23–4.
12. Dowell P, Peterson VJ, Zabriskie TM, Leid M. Ligand-induced peroxisome proliferator-activated receptor alpha conformational change. J Biol Chem. 1997;272:2013–20.
13. Kliewer SA, Sundseth SS, Jones SA, et al. Fatty acids and eicosanoids regulate gene expression through direct interaction with PPARα and PPARγ. Proc Natl Acad Sci USA. 1997;94:4318–23.
14. Forman BM, Chen J, Evans RM. Hypolipidemic drugs, polyunsaturated fatty acids and eicosanoids are ligands for PPARα and PPARγ. Proc Natl Acad Sci USA. 1997;94:4312–17.
15. Krey G, Braissant O, L'Horset F, et al. Fatty acids, eicosanoids and hypolipidemic agents identified as ligands of peroxisome proliferator activated receptors by CARLA. Mol Endocrinol. 1997;11:779–91.
16. Lee SS, Pineau T, Drago J, et al. Targeted disruption of the alpha isoform of the peroxisome proliferator-activated receptor gene in mice results in abolishment of the pleiotropic effects of peroxisome proliferators. Mol Cell Biol. 1995;15:3012–22.

15 The role of leukotrienes in rhinitis

P. H. HOWARTH

Allergic rhinitis is characterized by the symptoms of nasal itch, sneezing, rhinorrhoea and nasal stuffiness with, in addition in more severe and chronic disease, the development of mucosal oedema resulting in impaired sinus drainage, loss of sense of smell and altered eustachian tube function[1]. These symptoms and disruption of normal function are consequent upon the local release of mediators from activated cells within the nasal mucosa, through interactions with end-organ receptors. In this respect the nose differs from the lower respiratory tract in that symptom expression and disordered function are secondary to alterations in neural and vascular components and does not involve airway smooth muscle.

AIRWAY STRUCTURE – RELATIONSHIP TO SYMPTOM GENERATION

The two nasal air passages are structured medially by the nasal septum and laterally by a compliant nasal vestibule, anteriorly, and a bony cavum, posteriorly. The lateral wall of the bony component is lined by the turbinates. The state of engorgement of the venous sinusoids within these turbinates determines nasal airflow. The nasal vascular structure is complex, with arterioles beneath the basement membrane feeding subepithelial and glandular capillary networks which empty via cavernous sinusoids into draining venules. There are also arteriovenous (a-v) anastomoses diverting blood directly from the arterial to the venous system: it has been estimated that 60% of the total nasal blood flow is shunted through these a-v anastomoses. The superficial capillaries are fenestrated and can allow rapid exudation of protein-rich fluid into the nasal cavity, thereby contributing to nasal secretions. The cavernous sinuses, which comprise a plexus of venous capacitance vessels, are most dense in the inferior and middle turbinates. Their capacitance volume is under neural regulation, with intrinsic sympathetic tone limiting the sinusoidal capacity. The nasal vasculature can also be influenced by humoral factors, although their net effect may be complex dependent upon their site of action. This is illustrated by the potential effects of the prostanoid prostaglandin $(PG)E_2$, which may be produced by both activated eosinophils and by nasal epithelium. PGE_2 is 20 times more potent than adrenaline as a venoconstrictor[2] and would thus be anticipated to reduce nasal resistance and improve nasal airflow. However, PGE_2 is also a potent vasodilator of nasal resistance vessels[3] and would thus increase nasal blood flow, an action likely to increase nasal congestion and reduce nasal airflow. Thus, when a vasoactive mediator has the potential to exert opposing effects on differing components of the vascular system its site of release may determine its net influence.

In addition to the influence of humoral factors on the state of engorgement of the nasal venous tissue, such factors may also alter vascular permeability and, if enhancing plasma protein extravasation, contribute to the genesis of anterior nasal secretions. Superficial fenestrated capillaries are found beneath the basement membrane and around glands. An expansion of the interendothelial pore size allows unfiltered plasma to leak into the surrounding tissue by virtue of the intravascular hydrostatic pressure. The degree of extravasation will thus be determined by the active separation of the endothelial cells, the transendothelial pressure gradient and the magnitude of blood flow. Anterior nasal secretions will also be derived by discharge from the goblet and serous glands within the airway epithelium and from submucous and anterolateral deep glands within the airway submucosa. Glandular secretion is under neural regulation, predominantly parasympathetic. Thus stimulation of the afferent sensory neurones results in reflex glandular secretion[4,5]. In addition, stimulation of sensory nerve endings induces nasal discomfort/itch and also, with some stimuli, sneezing.

MUCOSAL INFLAMMATION AND POTENTIAL LIPID MEDIATOR GENERATION

Allergic rhinitis is characterized by mucosal inflammation with an accumulation of mast cells and eosinophils within the airway epithelium and leukocytes, in particular eosinophils, within the submucosa [6–8]. Nasal smears in seasonal rhinitis have also identified an increase in surface basophils[9,10]. These inflammatory cells all have the potential to generate lipid mediators and are in an activated state with ultrastructural features, on transmission electronmicroscopy, of degranulation. Because of the difficulty in obtaining sufficient tissue to study the release characteristics and lipid mediator profile of nasal mast cells, most information relating to airway mast cell behaviour is derived from lower airway mast cells. These cells generate leukotriene $(LTC)_4$ as their major 5-lipoxygenase (5-LO) product, at a concentration in the range of 5–30 $ng/10^6$ cells[11,12]. It is potentially possible that larger quantities may be generated and released in vivo, as studies on cultured human lung mast cell suggest that immunological LTC_4, LTB_4 and PGD_2 release from these cells, co-cultured with fibroblasts, is increased in comparison to recently dispersed and similarly activated cells[13]. It is likely that cytokines generated from the fibroblast support matrix, such as stem cell factor or nerve growth factor which promote mast cell growth and development, provide a microenvironment which influences 5-LO activity[14–16]. Basophils have the potential to generate comparable quantities of LTC_4[17,18], although, in contrast to human mast cells, the release of LTC_4 by basophils is inhibited by preincubation with corticosteroids[19].

Human eosinophils also contain lipoxygenase enzymes. The major 5-LO product of arachidonic acid cleavage from the cell phospholipid membrane is LTC_4, with lesser quantities of LTB_4 and LTD_4 also being synthesized[20]. Human eosinophils also possess 15-LO activity, generating in vitro 15-hydroxyeicosatetraenoic acid (15-HETE) and 5, 8 and 14, 15-diHETEs[21,22]. The ability of eosinophils to release LTC_4 is greatly enhanced if these cells have had prior exposure to a chemotactic stimulus such as LTB_4 or platelet activating factor (PAF), or are primed by cytokines such as interleukin

(IL)-3, IL-5 or granulocyte macrophage colony stimulating factor (GM-CSF)[23]. Human eosinophils can generate IL-3, IL-5 and GM-CSF, which may thus serve an autocrine function[24,25], and also contain the necessary acetyltransferase enzyme for PAF synthesis[23]. Immunological stimulation of eosinophils is, however, only associated with release of 5–10% of the synthesized PAF, the majority remaining cell-associated.

EVIDENCE FOR LIPID MEDIATOR RELEASE IN RHINITIS

Elevated levels of immunoreactive LTC_4/LTD_4 have been reported in nasal lavage fluid in both perennial allergic rhinitis[26] and in seasonal allergic rhinitis[27] (Figure 1). Elevated levels of LTs are also reported in nasal polyp tissue[28], a disease associated with tissue eosinophil recruitment.

The temporal release of LTs after allergen exposure has been explored using nasal allergen challenge and nasal lavage techniques. Creticos and colleagues demonstrated a dose-dependent increase in cysteinyl- (cys-) LTs, occurring within 10 minutes of challenge[29]. Although one subsequent study failed to confirm this finding[30], several others identified clear increments in LTC_4, LTD_4 and LTE_4 levels in nasal lavage fluid in association with the immediate nasal response[31–35] (Figure 2). Repeated nasal lavage sampling after allergen challenge has revealed a peak in LTC_4 immunoreactivity 5 minutes after challenge, which remains elevated at 30 minutes but returns to baseline levels by 60 minutes[33]. This peak in LTC_4 recovery and its subsequent decline is paralleled by subjective reporting of nasal obstruction, rhinorrhoea, nasal itch and sneeze. The specificity of these cys-LT changes for the allergic response has been suggested both by the lack of change in LTC_4 levels in nasal lavage in rhinitic subjects following

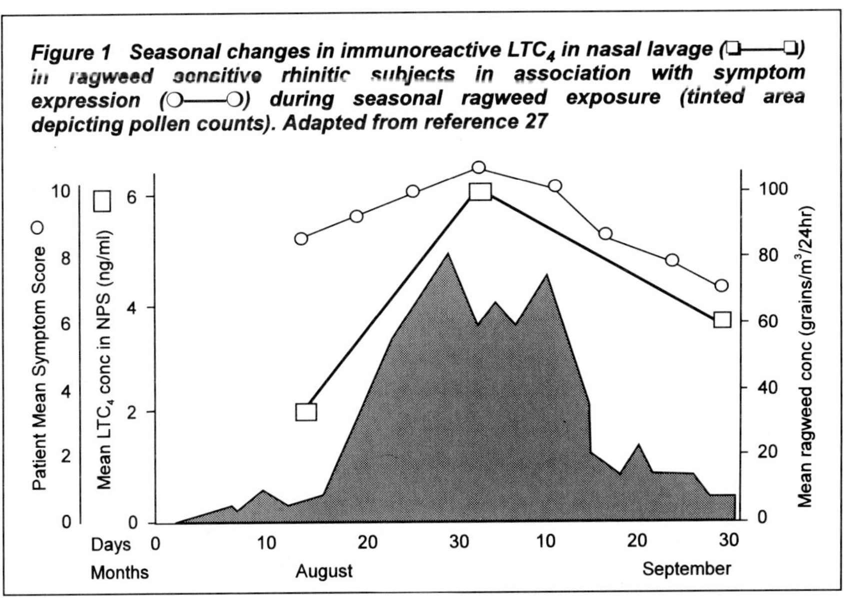

Figure 1   *Seasonal changes in immunoreactive LTC_4 in nasal lavage (□——□) in ragweed sensitive rhinitic subjects in association with symptom expression (○——○) during seasonal ragweed exposure (tinted area depicting pollen counts). Adapted from reference 27*

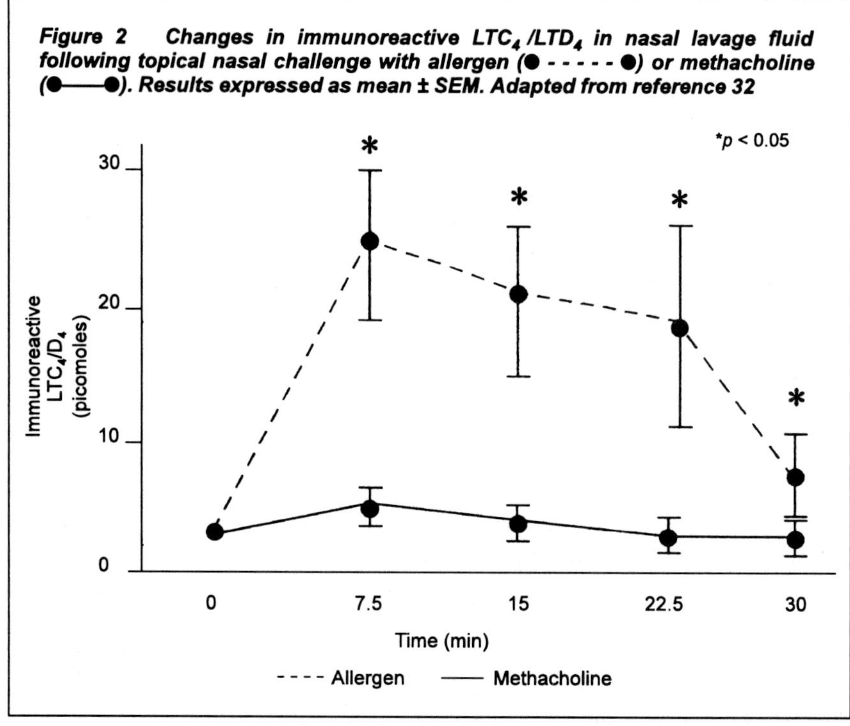

Figure 2   Changes in immunoreactive LTC$_4$/LTD$_4$ in nasal lavage fluid following topical nasal challenge with allergen (● - - - - - ●) or methacholine (●——●). Results expressed as mean ± SEM. Adapted from reference 32

saline, methacholine[32] or bradykinin[36] nasal challenge and, by the failure to detect elevations in non-atopic healthy volunteers following nasal allergen challenge[34]. It is not possible from studies such as these, however, to quantify the actual concentrations of LTs on the nasal mucosa as a considerable dilution factor occurs both on account of the lavage techniques (instillation of 5–10 ml saline between both nostrils) and on account of the challenge-induced changes both in glandular secretion and in vascular permeability with plasma protein extravasation. The one study attempting to overcome these limitations by adding radioactive albumin to the lavage fluid and correcting for dilution by the measurement of radioactivity in the recovered fluid was the one study which failed to detect an increase in the concentration of LTs in lavage fluid post challenge[30].

In addition to elevations in cys-LTs in nasal lavage following allergen challenge, immediate changes in LTs have also been described during the nasal response to cold air[37] and to nasal acetylsalicylic acid (ASA) challenge in aspirin-sensitive but not aspirin-insensitive rhinitic subjects or in healthy controls[38,39] (Figure 3). In contrast to the allergen-induced changes, which had resolved by 60 minutes after challenge, the ASA-induced changes in LTs were still evident at 60 minutes[39]. This increase in LTs in nasal lavage fluid was coincidental with the reporting by the sensitive patients of increased nasal secretion and nasal blockage, along with the identification of a significant increase in albumin levels in the lavage. Parallel measurement of PGE$_2$, PGF$_{2\alpha}$, PGD$_2$, 15-HETE

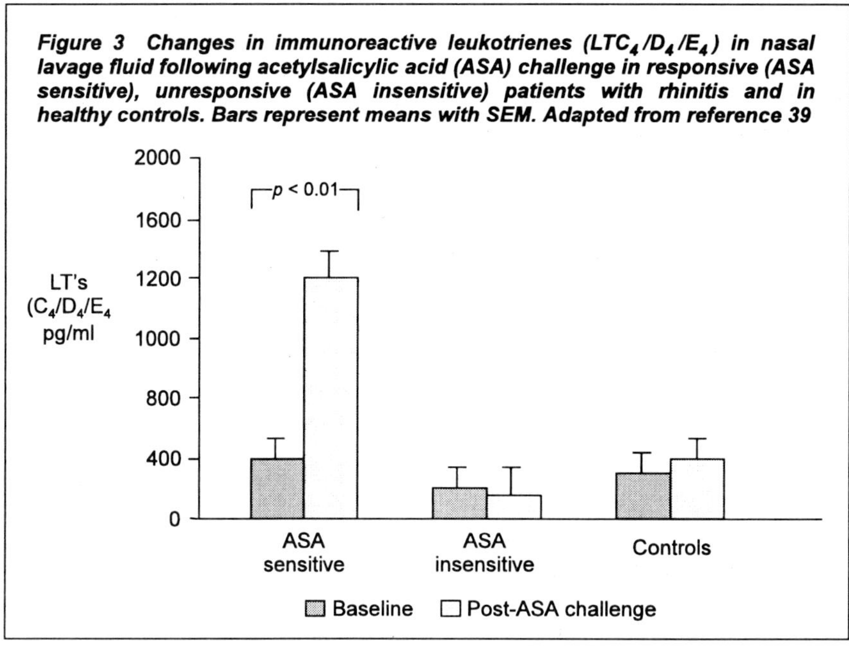

Figure 3   Changes in immunoreactive leukotrienes (LTC$_4$/D$_4$/E$_4$) in nasal lavage fluid following acetylsalicylic acid (ASA) challenge in responsive (ASA sensitive), unresponsive (ASA insensitive) patients with rhinitis and in healthy controls. Bars represent means with SEM. Adapted from reference 39

and LTB$_4$ has also been undertaken in association with saline and ASA challenge[39]. No change in LTB$_4$ levels is apparent despite the increase in LTC$_4$/LTD$_4$. Consistent with the inhibitory effect of ASA on cyclooxygenase enzymes, through its acetylation of the critical serine residue required for arachidonate binding by the enzyme, pretreatment induces a decrease in the concentration of PGE$_2$, PGF$_{2\alpha}$ and PGD$_2$ in the lavage fluid. These changes, with the exception of that for PGF$_2$, are, however, only present in the ASA-insensitive patients with no change in PGF$_{2\alpha}$ or PGD$_2$ lavage levels evident in ASA-sensitive patients. There is thus no simple relationship evident between cyclooxygenase inhibition and enhanced LT production as no change in lavage levels of peptide LTs was evident in the ASA-insensitive subjects.

Allergen-related increments in LTB$_4$ and 15-HETE have also been described during the immediate nasal response[40,41]. Repeated nasal lavage 4–12 h after challenge reveals a second increase in both LTB$_4$ and LTC$_4$[40,42]. There is no increase in tryptase or PGD$_2$ during these and later time points following nasal allergen challenge although nasal lavage histamine levels increase. As tryptase and PGD$_2$ are both mast cell-derived but histamine may be mast cell- or basophil-derived, these findings have been interpreted as indicating the relevance of basophil degranulation to the late nasal response. Consistent with this is the increased recovery of basophils but not mast cells in lavage during the late response and the identification that glucocorticosteroids inhibit the late rise in mediators in lavage, with the exception of LTB$_4$, without influencing the immediate increase[31,40,43]. The late changes in LTB$_4$ do not, however, appear specific for the challenge as late elevations in this arachidonic acid metabolite can be identified in non-atopic as well as atopic individuals following nasal allergen challenge.

RELEVANCE OF LIPID MEDIATORS TO RHINITIS SYMPTOMS

The nasal symptoms of itch, sneeze, rhinorrhoea and obstruction are determined by the neural and vascular effects of the mediators released during the allergic reaction and these mediators, along with cytokines, such as IL-1, IL-3, IL-4, IL-5, GM-CSF and tumour necrosis factor, will influence the cell recruitment and elaboration of the mucosal inflammatory reaction[44]. An understanding of the relevance of lipid mediators within the human model and in particular within the nose has been determined from topical challenge studies, from an understanding of the influence of these mediators on cell function and from investigation of the clinical effects of pharmacological intervention.

NASAL CHALLENGE STUDIES

Nasal insufflation studies identify that both LTC_4 and LTD_4 induce an increase in nasal airways resistance (NAR), as measured by rhinomanometry[33,45,46]. The nasal obstructive response to LTD_4 is more prolonged than that obtained with histamine when the two agonists are adjusted to produce a similar maximal response[45]. Studies to investigate effects of these two mediators within the nose have been undertaken both in asymptomatic grass pollen-sensitive subjects[33] and in house dust mite-sensitive perennial rhinitics[45]. In the former group, single dose challenges suggested that for a comparable maximal increase in nasal airways resistance (NAR) that LTC_4 was approximately 10 times more potent than histamine on a weight/volume basis (Figure 4). In contrast, the study in 14 patients with active rhinitis indicated that on a weight/volume basis LTD_4 was 5000 times more potent than histamine in achieving a 150% increase in NAR[45]. This increase in NAR was induced with a mean concentration of $2 \times 10^{-1.4}$ µg/ml. This diversity in comparative potency between active and inactive disease is paradoxically in contrast to the findings within the lower airways in which a much greater difference in potency has been recorded between LTs and histamine or methacholine in healthy controls than in asthma[47–49].

Nasal challenge studies with LTC_4 and LTD_4 have consistently identified no effect on nasal pruritus or sneezing, in contrast to the nasal effects of histamine. Although one study reported an acute nasal secretory response to nasal challenge with LTD_4[45], this was minimal in comparison to the effect of histamine and this has not been identified in other studies. It is possible that this small change in anterior nasal secretions could be accounted for by an increase in nasal vascular permeability. Laser Doppler flow studies within the nose have shown that, in addition to the effects of exogenously applied LTs on the state of engorgement of the venous sinusoids within the turbinates, that there is also a dose-related increase in nasal mucosal blood flow[46]. LTD_4 nasal challenge over a concentration range of 10–40 µm (approximately 5–20 µg), induced a 10–15% increase in mucosal blood flow. A similar change in mucosal blood flow was identified with the same concentrations of histamine applied topically to the nose in the same subjects. The findings of vasodilatation with LT administration within the nose confirm effects previously reported in the skin. Leukotrienes C_4, D_4 and E_4 all induce a local weal following intradermal injection, both in humans and in guinea-pigs[50–53]. Co-administration of

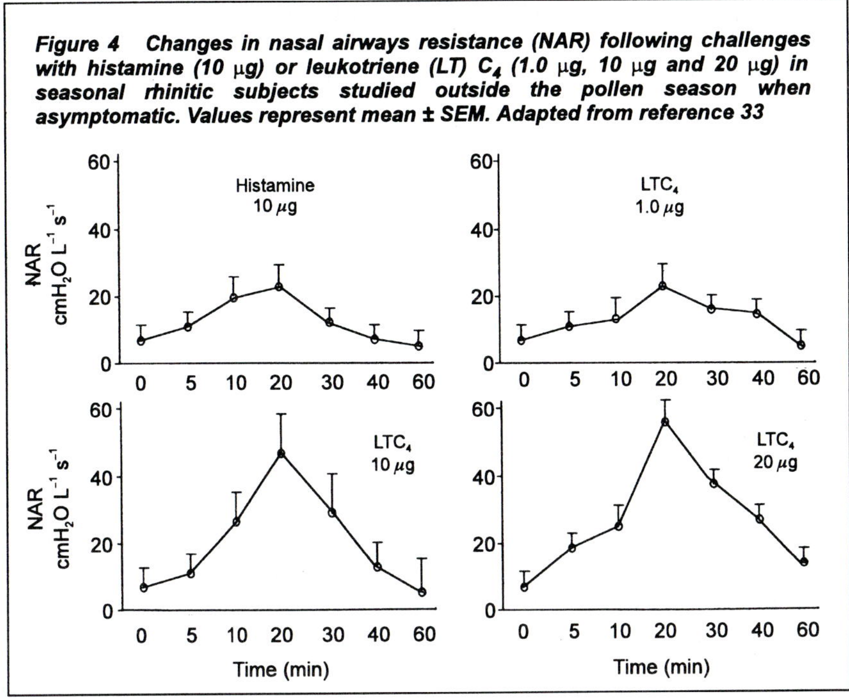

Figure 4   Changes in nasal airways resistance (NAR) following challenges with histamine (10 μg) or leukotriene (LT) C₄ (1.0 μg, 10 μg and 20 μg) in seasonal rhinitic subjects studied outside the pollen season when asymptomatic. Values represent mean ± SEM. Adapted from reference 33

PGE$_1$ or PGE$_2$ results in a synergistic inflammatory response[53] as a result of the vasodilator response of the prostanoids complementing the vasopermissive effects of the LTs.

INFLAMMATORY CELL RECRUITMENT

The LTs, particularly LTB$_4$, and the HETEs have potential relevance to the eosinophil airway recruitment which is evident in allergic rhinitis and to the neutrophil mucosal accumulation encountered in chronic rhinitis[8]. The intradermal injection of LTB$_4$ in human skin produces a small weal and flare response along with an accumulation of neutrophils at the site of administration[54]. Studies in vitro have identified that LTB$_4$ is a potent mediator of polymorphonucleocyte chemotaxis and aggregation as well as enhancing their state of activation, with increased lysozomal enzyme release and superoxide generation[55–57]. Although LTB$_4$ can induce an increase in vascular permeability per se, this effect is weak and is more pronounced in the presence of a vasodilator such as PGE$_2$. LTB$_4$ is also chemotactic for eosinophils[58]. The magnitude of eosinophil chemotaxis to LTB$_4$ is greater for cells primed by the cytokines IL-3, IL-5 and GM-CSF than with cytokine-naïve eosinophils[59].

The 15-LO arachidonate product 15-HETE, which has been identified in nasal lavage following allergen challenge[41], and 5,15-diHETE, 8,15-diHETE and 14,15-diHETE, which are generated by activated eosinophils, are also relevant to mucosal inflammation and cell activation in rhinitis (reviewed in 60). MonoHETE is weakly chemotactic for neutrophils, being 100 times less potent than LTB_4 in this respect, whereas 8,15- and 14,15-diHETE are without chemotactic activity in concentrations up to 10 µg/ml. More relevant, however, is the regulatory influence of these 15-LO arachidonic acid metabolites on eicosanoid production. 15-HETE potently inhibits cyclooxygenase and lipoxygenase enzymes and has been demonstrated to inhibit LTB_4 and 5-HETE generation from rabbit peritoneal neutrophils and PGI_2 generation by bovine aortic endothelial cells. Preincubation of human neutrophils with micromolar concentrations of 15-HETE activates the 15-LO pathway and inhibits the 5-LO pathway, thus reducing the synthesis of proinflammatory LTs. The generation of 15-HETE during the allergic airway response would thus serve to down-regulate the contribution of LTs to disease persistence.

INFLUENCE OF THERAPEUTIC INTERVENTION

An early study investigating the nasal protective effects of an oral LTD_4 antagonist L-649,923 failed to demonstrate any protective effect on the acute nasal response to allergen challenge[61]. This lack of effect, however reflects the lack of efficacy of this compound at the dose administered, rather than the non-involvement of LTs, since subsequent studies with a more potent LTD_4 antagonist in ragweed sensitive rhinitis[62] and a 5-LO inhibitor in a nasal allergen challenge setting[63] have both identified airway protective effects. The study with the oral LTD_4 antagonist, zafirlukast, identified in a placebo-controlled, double-blind, randomized trial design, a significant protective effect in ragweed sensitive rhinitis (Figure 5), in particular against the symptoms of stuffy nose, runny nose and sneezing during a 'day in the part' study over 2 days. In this study, four separate doses were assessed, (10 mg, 20 mg, 40 mg and 100 mg). The 20 mg and 40 mg doses both had significant effects but, for an unexplained reason, the 100 mg dose was no different in its efficacy to placebo. The study with the 5-LO inhibitor, zileuton, identified that the drug was biochemically effective within the nose, reducing LTB_4 and 5-HETE peaks post allergen challenge by 90.2% and 74% respectively in the absence of an effect on PGD_2 synthesis and release. Clinically there was a reduction in allergen-induced nasal congestion, but no significant influence on induced sneezes. A further study investigating the effect of a novel N-hydroxyurea 5-LO inhibitor (A-78773), which is 10 times as potent as zileuton, reported that single dose administration 5 h prior to nasal allergen insufflation protected over the 40 minute period of observation post challenge against both the challenge-related increase in nasal airways resistance, measured by active posterior rhinomanometry, and the increase in anterior nasal secretions[64]. No effect was identified on nasal itch or sneeze. In a subsequent nasal lavage study in the same subjects in association with nasal allergen challenge, A-78773 pretreatment significantly reduced the challenge-induced increments in total protein and albumin in lavage indicative of the involvement of LTs in allergic inflammation. The 5-LO inhibitor zileuton has also been shown to inhibit nasal symptom expression and the lavage increase in LTs associated with positive aspirin challenge in salicylate sensitive subjects[65]. No studies have investigated the

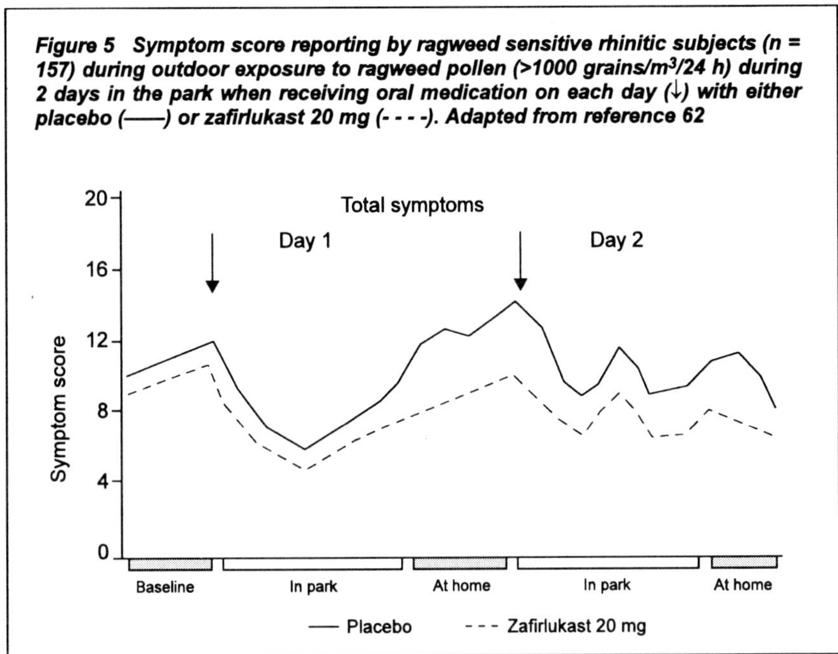

Figure 5 Symptom score reporting by ragweed sensitive rhinitic subjects (n = 157) during outdoor exposure to ragweed pollen (>1000 grains/m³/24 h) during 2 days in the park when receiving oral medication on each day (↓) with either placebo (——) or zafirlukast 20 mg (- - - -). Adapted from reference 62

influence of therapeutic intervention on the cellular components of inflammation in atopic airways disease. The identification that an LTD_4 antagonist, MK-571, partially inhibits allergen-induced eosinophil recruitment in the guinea-pig conjunctiva[66] does, however, suggest a potential for LT receptor antagonists or 5-LO inhibitors to modulate not only the plasma protein extravasation in allergic airway inflammation but also to influence tissue cell recruitment.

CONCLUSION

It is evident that LTs released in concert with mucosal inflammation contribute to rhinitis. Their release is evident in both naturally occurring and induced rhinitis and their involvement can be implicated both from challenge studies and from the limited information available from studies involving specific therapeutic intervention. With respect to symptom generation, their major effect appears to be vascular in inducing nasal congestion and plasma protein exudation. The generation of these mediators in the allergic response is thus an explanation for the lack of benefit of H_1-antihistamines in the treatment of nasal congestion, in contrast to the benefit of this mode of therapy in relieving nasal itch and sneeze and in reducing anterior nasal secretions[67,68]. Early intervention studies with LT receptor antagonists and 5-LO inhibitors confirm the theoretical involvement of LTs in nasal obstruction and also reveal a contribution from these eicosanoids in rhinorrhoea, enhanced vascular permeability and possibly also sneezing in the clinical setting, although not under controlled challenge conditions with respect to this later symptom. Future, more extensive studies with these and newly developing compounds will help to increase further the understanding of the role of lipid mediators in rhinitis.

References

1. Howarth PH. Allergic rhinitis: A rational choice of treatment. Resp Med.1989;83:179–88.
2. Bedwani J, Eccles R, Jones AS. The isolation of prostaglandin E from pig nasal mucosa. Clin Otolaryngol.1983;8:159–63.
3. Lung MA, Phipps RJ, Wang JCC, Widdicombe JG. Control of nasal vasculature and airflow resistance in the dog. J Physio.1984;349:535–51.
4. Baraniuk JN. Neural control of human nasal secretion. Pulm Pharmacol.1991;4:20–31.
5. Stjarne P, Lundblad L, Lundberg JM, Angaard A. Capsaicin and nicotine-sensitive afferent neurones and nasal secretion in healthy human volunteers and in patients with vasomolar rhinitis. Br J Pharmacol.1989;96:693–701.
6. Enerback L, Pipkorn U, Granerus G. Intraepithelial migration of nasal mucosal mast cells in hay fever. Int Arch Allergy Appl Immunol.1986;80:44–51.
7. Bentley AM, Jacobson MR, Cumberworth V, et al. Immunohistology of the nasal mucosa in seasonal allergic rhinitis: Increases in activated eosinophils and epithelial mast cells. J Allergy Clin Immunol.1992;89:877–83.
8. Montefort S, Feather IH, Wilson SJ, et al. The expression of leucocyte-endothelial adhesion molecules is increased in perennial allergen rhinitis. Am J Resp Cell Mol Biol.1992;7:393–8.
9. Otsuka H, Denburg JA, Dolovich J, et al. Heterogeneity of metachromatic cells in human nose: Significance of mucosal mast cells. J Allergy Clin Immunol.1985;76:695–702.
10. Okuda M, Ohtsuka H, Kawabori S. Studies of nasal surface basophilic cells. Ann Allergy.1985;54:69–71.
11. Peters SP, MacGlashan DW, Schulman ES, et al. Arachidonic acid metabolism in purified human lung mast cells. J Immunol.1984;132:1972–9.
12. MacGlashan DW, Schleimer RP, Peters SP, et al. Generation of leukotrienes by purified human lung mast cells. J Clin Invest.1982;70:747–51.
13. Levi-Schaffer F, Austen KF, Caulfield JP, Hein A, Gravallee PM, Stevens RL. Coculture of human lung-derived mast cells with mouse 3T3 fibroblasts: Morphology and IgE-mediated release of histamine, prostaglandin D_2 and leukotrienes. J Immunol.1987;139:494–500.
14. Levi-Schaffer FK, Austen K, Gravallee PM, Stevens RL. Coculture of interleukin 3-dependent mouse mast cells with fibroblasts results in a phenotypic change of the mast cells. Proc Natl Acad Sci USA.1986;83:6485–8.
15. Tsai M, Shih L-S, Newlands GEJ, et al. The rat c-kit ligand, stem cell factor, induces the development of connective tissue-type and mucosal mast cells in vivo, analysis bv anatomical distribution, histochemistry and protease phenotype. J Exp Med.1991;174:125–31.
16. Flint KC, Hudspith BN, Leung KBP, et al. IgE-dependent release of leukotriene C_4 and prostaglandin D_2 from human bronchoalveolar cells. Thorax.1985;40:716.
17. MacGlashan DW, Schleimer RP, Peters SP, et al. Comparative studies of human basophils and mast cells. Fed Proc.1983;42:2504–9.
18. MacGlashan DW, Peters SP, Warner JA, Lichtenstein LM. Characteristics of human basophil sulphidopeptide leukotriene release: Releasability defined as the ability of the basophil to respond to dineric cross-links. J Immunol.1986;136:2231–9.
19. Schleimer RP, Lichtenstein LM, Gillespie E. Inhibition of basophil histamine release by anti-inflammatory steroids. Nature.1981;292:454–5.
20. Weller PF, Lee CW, Foster DW, Corey EJ, Austen KF, Lewis RA. Generation and metabolism of 5-lipoxygenase pathway leukotrienes by human eosinophils: Predominant production of leukotriene C4. Proc Natl Acad Sci USA.1983;80:7626–30.
21. Turk J, Maas RL, Brash AR, Roberts LJ, Oates JA. Arachidonic acid 15-lipoxygenase products from human eosinophils. J Biol Chem.1982;257:7068.
22. Henderson WR, Harley JB, Fanci AS. Arachidonic acid metabolism in normal and

hypereosinophilic syndrome human eosinophils: Generation of leukotrienes B_4, C_4, D_4 and 15-lipoxygenase products. Immunology.1984;51:679.

23. Frigas E, Gleich GJ. The role of eosinophils. In: Lessoff MH, Lee TH, Kemeny DM, editors. Allergy: an International Textbook. Chichester: Wiley, 1987;137–55.

24. Kita H, Ohnishi T, Okuba Y, Weiler D, Abrams JS, Gleich GJ. Granulocyte macrophage colony-stimulating factor and interleukin-3 release from human peripheral blood eosinophils and neutrophils. J Exp Med.1991;174:745–8.

25. Desreumaux P, Janin A, Colombel JF, et al. Interleukin-5 messenger RNA expression in the intestine mucosa of patients with coeliac disease. J Exp Med.1992;175:293–6.

26. Knani J, Campbell A, Enander I, Peterson CG, Michel RB, Bousquet J. Indirect evidence of nasal inflammation assessed by titration of inflammatory mediators and enumeration of cells in nasal secretions of patients with chronic rhinitis. J Allergy Clin Immunol.1992;90:880–9.

27. Volovitz B, Osur SL, Berstein JM, Ogra PL. Leukotriene C_4 release in upper respiratory mucosa during natural exposure to ragweed in ragweed-sensitive children. J Allergy Clin Immunol.1988;82:414–18.

28. Jung TTK, Juhn SK, Hwang D, et al. Prostaglandins, leukotrienes and other arachidonic acid metabolites in nasal polyps and nasal mucosa. Laryngoscope.1987;97:184–9.

29. Creticos PS, Peters SP, Adkinson NF Jr, et al. Peptide leukotriene release after antigen challenge in patients sensitive to ragweed. N Engl J Med.1984;310:1626–30.

30. Bisgaard H, Robinson C, Romeling F, Mygind N, Church MK, Holgate ST. Leukotriene C_4 and histamine in early allergic reaction in the nose. Allergy.1988;43:219–27.

31. Pipkorn U, Proud D, Lichtenstein LM, et al. Effect of short term systemic glucocorticoid treatment on human nasal mediator release after allergen challenge. J Clin Invest.1987;80:957–61.

32. Shaw RJ, Fitzharris P, Cromwell I, Wardlaw AJ, Kay AB. Allergen-induced release of sulphidopeptide leukotrienes (SRS-A) and LTB_4 in allergic rhinitis. Allergy.1985;40:1–6.

33. Miadonna A, Tedeschi A, Leggieri E, et al. Behaviour and clinical relevance of histamine and leukotrienes C_4 and B_4 in grass-pollen-induced rhinitis. Am Rev Resp Dis.1987;136:357–62.

34. Ophir C, Fink A, Eliraz A, Tabachnik E, Bentwich Z. Allergen-induced leukotriene production by nasal mucosa and peripheral blood leucocytes. Arch Otolaryngol Head Neck Surg.1988;114:522–4.

35. Kojima T, Asakura K. The study of chemical mediators in patients with allergic rhinitis. 2) Histamine, leukotriene and kinins in the nasal secretion during dual phase response. Nippon Jibinkoka Gakkai Kaiho.1991;94:366–76.

36. Brunnee T, Nigam S, Kunkel G, Baumgarten CR. Nasal challenge studies with bradykinin: Influence upon mediator generation. Clin Exp Allergy.1991;21:425–31.

37. Togias AG, Nacclerio RM, Peters SP, et al. Local generation of sulfidopeptide leukotrienes upon nasal provocation with cold, dry air. Am Rev Resp Dis.1986;133:1133–7.

38. Ferreri NR, Howland WC, Stevenson DD, Spiegelberg HL. Release of leukotrienes, prostaglandins and histamine into nasal secretions of aspirin-sensitive asthmatics during reaction to aspirin. Am Rev Resp Dis.1988;137:847–54.

39. Picardo C, Ramis I, Rosello J, et al. Release of peptide leukotriene into nasal secretions after local instillation of aspirin in aspirin-sensitive asthmatic patients. Am Rev Resp Dis.1992;145:65–9.

40. Freeland HS, Pipkorn U, Schleimer RP, Bascom R, Lichtenstein LM, Naclerio RM, Peters SP. Leukotriene B_4 as a mediator of early and later reactions to antigen in humans: The effect of systemic glucocorticoid treatment in vivo. Am Rev Resp Dis.1989;83:634–42.

41. Ramis I, Catafan JR, Serra J, Bulbena O, Picardo C, Gelpi E. In vivo release of 15-HETE and other arachidonic acid metabolites in nasal secretions during early allergic reactions. Prostaglandins.1991;42:411–20.

42. Naclerio RM, Proud D, Togias AG, et al. Inflammatory mediators in late antigen-induced rhinitis. New Engl J Med.1985;313:65–70.

43. Bascom R, Wachs M, Naclerio RM, Pipkorn U, Galli SJ, Lichtenstein LM. Basophil influx occurs after nasal challenge: Effects of topical corticosteroid pretreatment. J Allergy Clin Immunol.1988;81:580–9.

44. Howarth PH, Bradding P, Quint D, Redington AE, Holgate ST. Cytokines and airway inflammation. Ann NY Acad Sci; in press.

45. Okuda M, Watase T, Mezawa A, Liu C-M. The role of leukotriene D_4 in allergic rhinitis. Ann Allergy.1988;60:537–40.

46. Bisgaard H, Olsson P, Bende M. Effect of leukotriene D_4 on nasal mucosal blood flow, nasal airways resistance and nasal secretions in humans. Clin Allergy.1986;16:289–97.

47. Weiss JW, Drazen JM, Coles, et al. Bronchoconstrictor effects of leukotriene C in humans. Science.1982;216:196–8.

48. Barnes NC, Piper PJ, Costello JF. Comparative effects of inhaled leukotriene C_4, leukotriene D_4 and histamine in normal human subjects. Thorax.1984;39:500.

49. Adelroth E, Morris MM, Hargreave FE, O'Byrne PM. Airway responsiveness to leukotriene C_4 and D_4 and to methacholine in patients with asthma and normal controls. N Engl J Med.1986;315:480–4.

50. Soter NA, Lewis RA, Corey EJ, Austen KF. Locals effects of synthetic leukotrienes (LTC_4, LTD_4, LTE_4 and LTB_4) in human skin. J Invest Dermatol.1983;80:115–19.

51. Bisgaard H. Vascular effects of leukotriene D_4 in human skin. J Invest Dermatol.1987;88:109–14.

52. Drazen JM, Austen KF, Lewis RA, et al. Comparative airway and vascular activities of leukotrienes C-1 and D in vivo and in vitro. Prox Natl Acad Sci USA.1980;77:4354–8.

53. Peck MJ, Piper PJ, Williams TJ. The effect of leukotrienes C_4 and D_4 on the microvasculature of guinea-pig skin. Prostaglandins.1981;21:315–21.

54. Camp RDR, Coutts AA, Greaves MW, Kay AB, Walport MJ. Responses of human skin to intradermal injection of leukotrienes C_4, D_4 and B_4. Br J Pharmacol.1982;75:168–71.

55. Ford-Hutchinson AW, Bray MA, Doig MV, Shipley ME, Smith MJH. Leukotriene B_4 is a potent chemokinetic and aggregating substance released from polymorphonuclear leucocytes. Nature.1980;286:64–5.

56. Palmblad J, Malmsten CL, Uden AM, Radmark O, Engstedt L, Samuelsson B. Leukotriene B_4 is a potent and stereospecific stimulator of neutrophil chemotaxis and adherence. Blood.1981;58:658–61.

57. Ford-Hutchinson AW, Bray MA, Shipley ME, Doig MV, Smith JPH. Leukotriene B_4 is a potent mediator of leucocyte function released from polymorphonuclear leucocytes. Int J Immunopharmacol.1986;2:232–7.

58. Nagy L, Lee TH, Gretyl EJ, Pickett WS, Kay AB. Complement receptor enhancement and chemotaxis of human neutrophils and eosinophils by leukotrienes and other lipoxygenase products. Clin Exp Immunol.1982;47:541–7.

59. Warringa RAJ, Koenderman L, Kok PIM, Kreukniet J, Bruijnzeel PLB. Modulation and induction of eosinophil chemotaxis by granulocyte-macrophage colony stimulating factor and interleukin-3. Blood.1991;77:2694–700.

60. Henderson WR. Products of 12- and 15- lipoxygenase. In: Henson PM, Murphy RC, editors. Mediators of Inflammatory Process. Amsterdam: Elsevier, 1989;45–75.

61. Flowers BK, Proud D, Kagey-Sabotka A, Lichtenstein LM, Naclerio RM. The effect of a leukotriene antagonist on the early response to antigen. Otolaryngol Head Neck Surg.1990;102:219–24.

62. Donnelly A, Glass M, Muller B, et al. The leukotriene D_4 receptor antagonist, ICI 204:219, relieves symptoms of acute seasonal allergic rhinitis symptoms. Am J Resp Crit Care Med.1995;151:1734–9.

63. Knapp HR. Reduced allergen-induced nasal congestion and leukotriene synthesis with an orally active 5-lipoxygenase inhibitor. New Engl J Med.1990;327:1745–8.

64. Howarth PH, Harrison K, Lau L. The influence of 5-lipoxygenase inhibition in allergic rhinitis. Int Arch Allergy Appl Immunol.1995;107:423–4.

65. Fischer AR, Rosenberg MA, Lilly CM, et al. Direct evidence for a role of the mast cell in the nasal response to aspirin in aspirin-sensitive asthma. J Allergy Clin Immunol,1994;94:1046–56.

66. Chan C-C, McKee K, Tagari P, Chee P, Ford-Hutchinson A. Eosinophil-eicosanoid interactions: Inhibition of eosinophil chemotaxis in vivo by an LTD_4-receptor antagonist. Eur J Pharmacol.1990;191:273–80.

67. Howarth PH, Emanuel MB, Holgate ST. Astemizole, a potent histamine H_1-receptor

antagonist: effect in allergic rhinoconjunctivitis, on antigen and histamine induced skin weal responses and relationship to serum levels. Br J Clin Pharmacol.1984;18:1–8.
68. Howarth PH, Holgate ST. Comparative trial of two non-sedative H_1-antihistamines, terfenadine and astemizole for hay fever. Thorax.1984;39:668–72.

Index